TARGET YOUR FAT SPOTS

how to banish your bulges

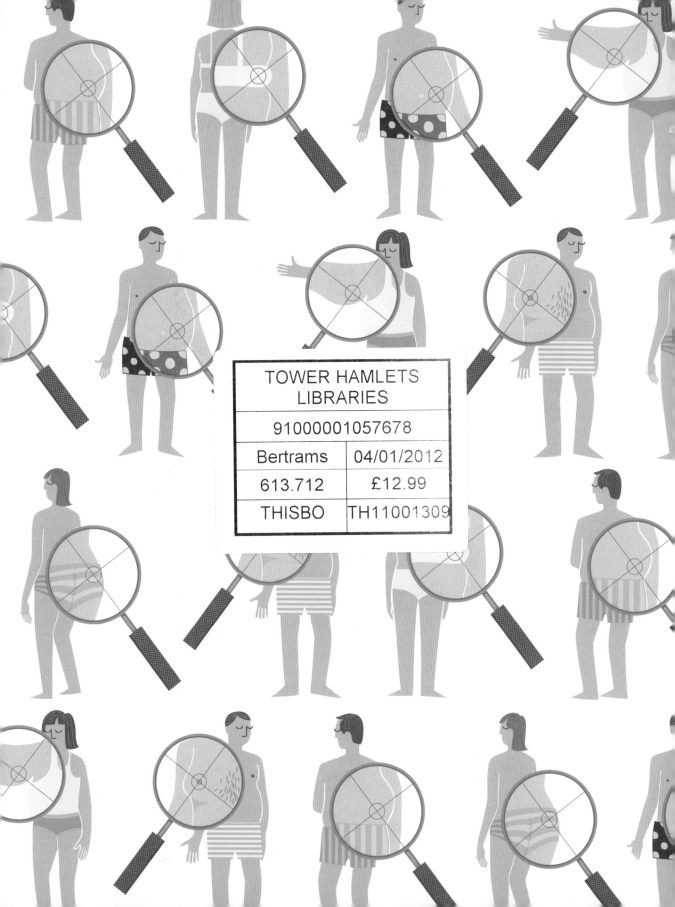

TARGET YOUR FAT SPOTS

how to banish your bulges

MAX TOMLINSON ND

Quadrille
PUBLISHING

To my wife, my wonderful family and my dear friends

FOREWORD

Naturopathy is my life's passion, and complementary medicine (CAM) is my long and abiding obsession. Complementary medicine is here to stay, and I am proud of the small role I have played in helping it to become recognised for what it is: a highly effective way to become and stay healthy.

This book is based on the very successful fat spot reduction programme I run in my London clinic. For over 24 years I have been helping my clients become healthy and lose weight, and fat spot reduction is the pinnacle of my professional achievement – the end result of years of study and experimentation. I can't supply all my evidence in the form of peer-reviewed, double blind, placebo-controlled clinical trials while pushing the boundaries of understanding how hormones influence fat deposits, but what I can do here is introduce a new approach to losing stubborn fat and regaining glowing health.

I developed my spot fat reduction programme to target the weird, disproportionate fat deposits I was seeing in my clients: men with a reasonable overall body shape, but with excess fat stored on their stomachs and lower backs; young women who had tried rigorous diets and exercise regimes to get rid of a big bottom, for example, only to lose weight from their chests and faces; and menopausal women who tended to accumulate fat on their stomachs and under their upper arms as they aged. I spent years looking for links in research literature that would provide clues to help me. Then advances in a new type of laboratory testing, called functional medicine testing, gave me the breakthrough I needed and helped me to see a way forwards.

This book has two crystal-clear aims. The first is to help you get rid of any unsightly fat spots that you have lovingly created. I want you to get healthy, bust your fat spots once and for all, lose some weight and feel great about yourself. The programmes I describe will help you to restore a more balanced and healthy look to your body. You will also learn how to detox your diet and lifestyle to rebalance what can only be described as a topsy-turvy toxic world of sugary, fatty reasons to put on weight. I will teach you to look after yourself in the present, the 'here and now', actively preventing age-related illness and ugly fat spot weight gain.

My second aim is 'no rubbish'. This book is simple, easy to use and free of excess chapters or page fillers. My explanations are direct and my tools are effective. I have the knowledge to help you succeed if you have the time and the inner strength to listen, digest and act on my advice. I won't be giving you endless lists on what to do or what not to do; instead I hope to inspire you to use your intelligence and take the initiative to follow my plan effectively.

Take the challenge. The old saying that action makes traction applies here. Step up, embrace change and set your sights on a new, vital, proud **YOU**.

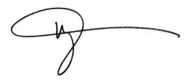

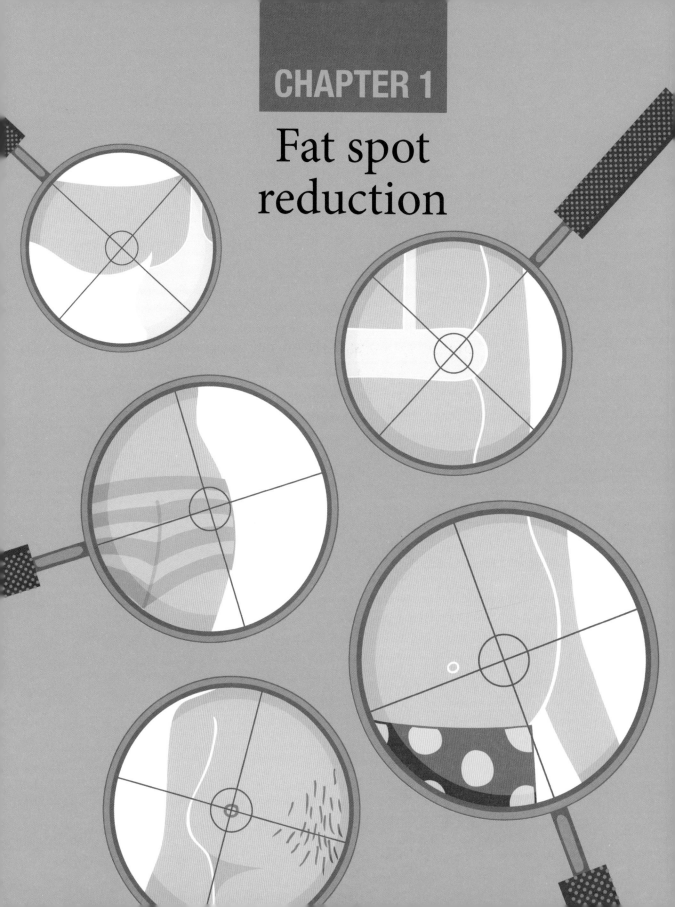

CHAPTER 1

Fat spot reduction

Welcome to chapter one. In this chapter I introduce the concept of fat spot reduction and explain my reasoning as to why we accumulate fat in certain areas of the body. I cover six main fat spots in this book; these are the areas that I see daily in my clinic and which I can help you with:

★ Love handles – the stuff that bulges over the back and sides of your jeans ♀♂
★ Stomach fat – a not so yummy tummy ♀♂
★ Bra bulge fat – the fat that makes it hard to get a bra to fit ♀
★ Bingo wings – the dangling fat hanging from your upper arms ♀
★ Big thighs and butt – fat thighs and a big bottom ♀
★ Moobs – one for the boys. Man boobs ♂

Interested now? Have you got one, or even two, troublesome fat spots of your own? Do you want to sort your weight and body shape out once and for all? Time, then, to find out why you have your fat spot and learn how to drop the weight and correct your body shape.

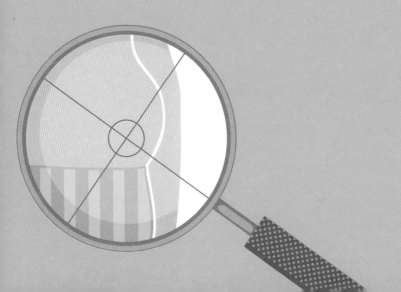

♀ = female
♂ = male

Fat spot reduction **WHAT IT IS NOT**

Before we go any further, we need to be very clear about my definition of fat spot reduction. It is NOT about exercising a specific part of your body in the gym every day in a vain attempt to lose weight from that specific area.

You may, for instance, be doing lots of sit-ups in the hope of achieving a trim stomach. I suggest you **STOP RIGHT NOW.** I have not found any evidence in my clinic, in the latest scientific literature or in the gym that supports the idea that you can exercise weight off a fat spot. I want to state at the outset that I believe there is no way you can effectively or significantly reduce fat surrounding the muscles on your stomach by just working your stomach muscles; muscle and fat are two completely different tissues. If you are indulging in this exercise madness, all you will get is a toned, but still fat, stomach.

In the same way, I have seen young women with large thighs take to the exercise bikes in the gym with great dedication, only to end up with even bigger thighs after months of sweat and tears. If we look briefly at why this is so for those young women, the reason is that the female hormone, oestrogen, promotes the laying down of fat on the thighs of younger women as fuel for a potential pregnancy. This fat spot is therefore perfectly natural and very feminine when in proportion (as women age and their oestrogen levels fall, the fat on their legs and bottom migrates onto their stomachs).

'It is **NOT** about exercising a specific part of your body in the gym every day in an attempt to lose weight from that specific area'

TO ACHIEVE TARGETED FAT LOSS, YOU NEED TO FOCUS ON THE REASON FOR FAT BEING LAID DOWN IN A SPECIFIC AREA OF YOUR BODY.

Fat spot reduction **WHAT IT IS**

My fat spot reduction programme is all about you achieving the kind of specific, targeted weight loss that no other dieting method, exercise regime or course of supplements can accomplish.

Based on my years of clinical experience and laboratory testing, I have come to the conclusion that one of the main reasons so many people have stubborn or problem fat areas is due to **IMBALANCES IN THEIR HORMONES**.

A multitude of processes in the body are co-ordinated by hormones that regulate and balance the workings of internal organs and cells. Some hormones have long-term effects, such as the human growth hormone (HGH), which controls how we grow, and the sex hormones that cause the changes that happen at puberty. Other hormones have shorter-term effects, such as insulin, which regulates the increased glucose that circulates in the blood every time we eat.

Some body builders and the occasional misguided athlete take hormones (steroids) to build muscle and some of them end up quite large and misshapen. So we know that hormones have a profound effect on the body and can build really big muscular bodies.

Hormones also govern where we store fat; women and men tend to store fat on different parts of their bodies (men on their guts, women on their butts). More generally, women hold fat in a concentrated layer, called subcutaneous fat, directly under their skin, while men store fat inside the abdomen near their internal organs.

'Small hormonal imbalances can have major consequences for our bodies'

UNBALANCED HORMONES IN YOUR BODY

The basic premise of this book is that just as steroid hormones build muscle, other hormones, when unbalanced, can build unwanted fluid and fat stores on areas such as your hips, legs and stomach. I read an interesting piece of research recently on the effects of sleep deprivation on levels of the hormone insulin. Losing as little as an hour and a half of sleep a night is enough to raise insulin levels in the body. That does not sound like a major issue until you realise that insulin promotes fat deposition on the stomach. So small hormonal imbalances can have major consequences for our bodies.

The question you must be asking now is why and how do your hormones become unbalanced. You will have to read on to get the full story, but essentially hormonal imbalance is caused by a combination of poor diet, lifestyle factors such as stress and environmental pollution and lack of effective exercise.

What exactly is **INVOLVED?**

Restoring your body to its correct hormonal balance is an essential element in reducing your fat spot. The really good news is that over the past 20 years advancements in functional medicine laboratory testing and targeted nutritional supplements have given me a greater understanding of which hormones in the body may be unbalanced, and how to rebalance them. These same advances have also given me the tools to help combat fat storage at specific sites on the body. You are living in the perfect moment to tackle your fat spot.

WHAT IS FUNCTIONAL MEDICINE TESTING?

Functional medicine is best defined as personalised (specific to the individual) medicine that deals primarily with the prevention of disease. Practitioners of this new form of medicine strive to address the underlying causes of an illness rather than just modifying or calming any obvious signs and symptoms. Functional medicine practitioners use modern scientific functional medicine testing to analyse exactly what is wrong with their patients. In my London clinic I use these accurate blood, urine and saliva laboratory tests to throw a spotlight on how well a client's particular hormonal gland, body system or organ is functioning. With functional medicine testing I get a clear snapshot of my client's health before it degrades further and a disease develops. This enables me to intervene with natural medicines to support a less-than-optimal functioning organ or a tired or under-nourished gland in a client's body. An example of this would be the combination of vitamins, minerals and medicinal herbs that I would give to a client to support his or her thyroid if one of these particular laboratory tests revealed that the client's thyroid was not functioning 100 per cent efficiently.

'I have developed some simple, wonderfully effective questionnaires that will enable you to assess accurately your own health status in relation to your specific fat spot'

As laboratory tests are expensive and can be hard to access, I have developed some simple, wonderfully effective questionnaires in chapter three that will enable you to accurately assess your own health status in relation to your specific fat spot. Be assured that although the process of testing in this book may use different methods from the lab tests I use in clinic, we will still get to the root of your problem and tackle your fat spot effectively. It has taken me over ten years to refine each questionnaire and I have used them on countless clients. They analyse the most common symptoms representing the particular hormonal dysfunction that is creating your fat spot.

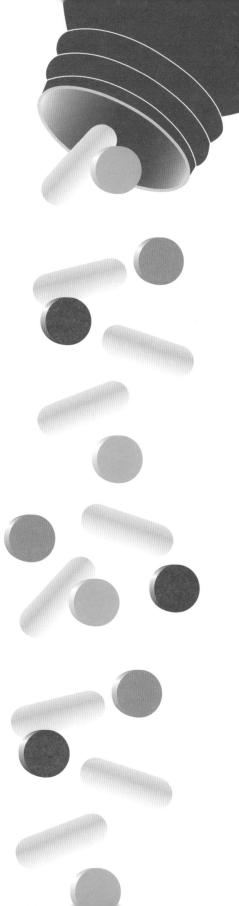

WHAT ARE TARGETED NUTRITIONAL SUPPLEMENTS?

Most of us are familiar with vitamin and mineral supplements, and may waste lots of our hard-earned money each year on a medicine cabinet full of the latest must-have 'miracle' or celebrity endorsed supplements. We tend to pick supplements randomly, not knowing whether they really benefit our bodies or not.

What you will discover in this book is that nutritional science and the use of supplementation has advanced to the point where it is now possible to guarantee that a specific combination of nutrients in a supplement will have a defined improvement on your health: herbs, vitamins, minerals and other natural compounds can all be combined to create a positive healing effect in your body. A good example of this is the very effective combination of tyrosine, kelp, B complex vitamins and copper that I use to combat sluggish thyroid function, which is associated with a bra fat spot.

I have been at the forefront of this new nutritional health science for many years and my clients reap the benefits daily. By carefully following my recommendations in this book, you can claim the benefits too.

While correcting your hormonal imbalance is vital, it is by no means sufficient on its own to tackle your fat spot. What I prescribe is a three-pronged approach that includes targeted exercise and corrective eating in addition to taking specific supplements. These three approaches all work in synergy to sort out your fat spot problem.

TAILORED EXERCISE

If you panic at the thought of having to sweat it out in the gym to improve your body shape, relax. I am a firm believer in 'clever', not hard, exercise, by which I mean following carefully tailored, or planned, exercise routines. In fact, as I mentioned before, some forms of intense exercise may actually make your fat spot grow larger (see box, below left).

A friend of mine, who is a top celebrity trainer in New York, says that the best exercise you do is the exercise you do; it is time to put some of the joy back into exercise. I want you to want to exercise, to see the benefits and marvel at the changes to your body shape that targeted exercise can bring. Quite simply, I will ask you to follow an effective, professionally designed exercise programme that works in combination with my healthy eating plan and specific nutritional supplements to help you shed your fat spot.

If all this sounds good and easy, then let's get real: you will need to do the exercise to make a difference to your fat spot.

A WORD OF CAUTION

Some forms of intense exercise may increase your fat spot. For example, if you have fat thighs and a big bottom, you may want to jump on an exercise bike to lose the weight, but you will end up with super-sized thighs as your thigh muscles grow and fat is deposited nearby to fuel the exercise. And if you run for longer than 45 minutes, you may be adding to your stomach fat, as the body releases cortisol in response to the stress of running, which in turn slows your thyroid down. Perhaps you have already experienced this?

WHY CHANGE WHAT I EAT?

Natural therapists like me work to change the unhealthy, damaging and fattening way that a lot of us habitually eat. One of the common consequences of changing your poor eating patterns is a return to a healthy weight and an improved overall shape.

I have tailored the majority of my corrective eating plans for fat spot reduction in chapter five around the supremely healthy Mediterranean cuisine, with additional specific changes that apply to each fat spot. You are about to embark on a tasty, healthy and varied culinary experience, which also focuses on reducing the amount of meat, white bread, sugar and salt that you will eat. None of the dietary changes I will ask you to make are too hard, and they will all benefit your overall health and wellbeing.

Incidentally, you may notice that I avoid using the word 'diet'. I do this on purpose because the word has been hijacked by the weight-loss industry and now carries connotations of restrictive eating and dramatic weight loss (that is ultimately unsustainable).

My eating plans are not about drastic weight loss, they are about changing the way you eat so that you live a healthier, more active and more fulfilled life. I hope that you will be so inspired by this new way of eating that you will never go back to your old ways, which is a good thing since your new diet will also help you keep your fat spot away – permanently.

So fat spot reduction is all about losing fat from a specific fat storage area on your body by correcting your personal hormonal imbalance with nutritional supplements, improving your overall health by following a prescribed way of healthy eating and using tailored exercise to reshape your body.

Over the next few pages I go into detail about which hormones affect which parts of the body. Take your time and read carefully. I want you to understand fully the reasons for your current weight gain.

The **OXFORD DICTIONARY** defines the word 'diet' primarily as:

diet[1] (noun) The kinds of food that a person, animal, or community habitually eats.

The **CAMBRIDGE DICTIONARY** defines the word 'diet' as:

diet[1] (daɪet) *n.* **1.** The food and drink usually eaten or drunk by a person or group.

No mention of weight loss here!

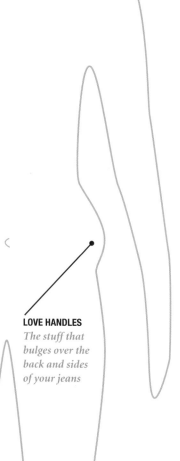

LOVE HANDLES

The stuff that bulges over the back and sides of your jeans

The six **FAT SPOTS**

It's now time to get personal and find out what the different fat spots reveal about your own body. These are simple summaries of the main reasons for your particular fat spot (I expand on the specific hormones and what they do in chapter two).

LOVE HANDLES ♀♂

If you have an excessive amount of fat on the area above your hips, this tendency indicates that you have an **INSULIN** problem and your body needs help handling the carbohydrates and sugars in your diet.

The carbohydrates in foods such as rice are broken down by your digestive system into a simple sugar, glucose, which circulates in the blood and provides each and every body cell with fuel to power your days and nights. Under normal conditions the hormone insulin regulates your blood glucose levels (the amount of glucose in your bloodstream) and diverts any excess glucose into the liver and muscles to be stored as glycogen, a store of fuel for future energy needs.

However, modern sugar-rich diets often lead to a condition called insulin resistance, whereby insulin does not manage blood sugars correctly or store glucose properly. This leads to elevated insulin levels, as the body produces more insulin in an attempt to control the excess glucose in the bloodstream. High insulin levels cause fat to be deposited in fat cells. Long-term insulin resistance is potentially dangerous and may lead to adult-onset, or type 2, diabetes and polycystic ovaries. It may also put you at risk of heart disease.

DID YOU KNOW...

Sugar is a significant part of our diet, however much we try to avoid it. On average, we each consume 30 teaspoons of sugar every day. Naturopaths state that part of the problem is that many of us do not realise we are eating hidden sugars. Sugar can be present in surprisingly large quantities in food that you would otherwise regard as healthy. Baked beans, orange juice and flavoured yoghurts are all examples of foods that contain hidden sugars.

STOMACH FAT ♀♂

If you have an excessive amount of fat on your stomach area, this suggests that you have a problem with your adrenal glands and **CORTISOL** production.

Our adrenal glands produce the hormones adrenaline and cortisol when we are faced with stressful situations. Adrenaline initiates a primitive reaction called the 'fight or flight' response: it raises your blood pressure, drives blood to the muscles and the brain so you can react quickly, raises your heart rate and speeds up your breathing. It also increases the flow of glucose, protein and fat into the bloodstream to cope with the crisis and fuel your muscles in case you need to run away fast. This is fine for short bursts of stress or activity; the damage occurs if you experience long-term stress, as cortisol, rather than adrenaline, is released. High levels of cortisol over a long period of time can cause accelerated ageing, stomach fat deposition, loss of muscle and bone mass, heart disease and even damage to brain cells. My interest in stomach fat began when I learned that it is strongly associated with obesity-related diseases such as heart attacks and stroke.

In addition, sustained high glucose levels in the bloodstream cause high levels of insulin to be released, which results in excess glucose being stored as fat (left). So being stressed can make you unhealthy and fat! This is one fat spot we all need to take seriously.

DID YOU KNOW...

It is estimated that every year millions of people across Europe and the United States find themselves under so much stress at work that they become sick, and this accounts for a huge amount of lost working days a year. Given that work is just one source of stress, the sheer magnitude of the problem of adrenal stress in modern society is very worrying indeed.

Adrenal fatigue is an umbrella term for a list of non-specific symptoms: tiredness, irritability, feeling light-headed upon standing, low sex drive, difficulty concentrating, poor sleep and problems with digestion. Standard medical hormonal blood tests for adrenal function may come back as 'normal', even though a patient's adrenal glands are performing sub-optimally.

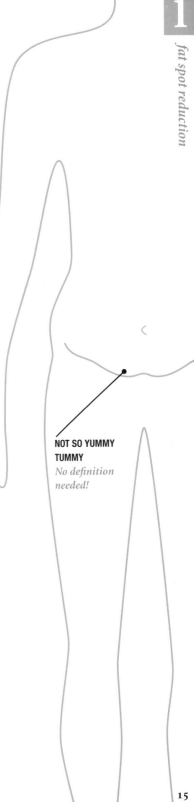

NOT SO YUMMY TUMMY
No definition needed!

BRA BULGE FAT

The fat that makes it hard to get a bra to fit

BRA BULGE FAT ♀

If you have an excessive amount of fat on your upper back, with fat bulging out of the sides of your bra, you may well have a sluggish thyroid. This gland secretes two hormones, **THYROXINE (T4)** and **TRIIODOTHYRONINE (T3)**, which govern your metabolic rate – the rate at which you burn up calories from the food you eat.

We all know people who can eat anything they like and not put on any weight. They have excellent thyroid function. The opposite is true of someone who eats mainly lettuce leaves and doesn't lose any weight. Hypothyroidism (low thyroid function) is a growing problem, and is largely undiagnosed by modern medicine due to the limited nature of the standard medical hormonal blood tests that are usually carried out. Hypothyroidism can cause bra fat deposits, overall weight gain, fatigue, depression, low body temperature, constipation, decreased memory and poor concentration. Complete my questionnaire in chapter three and do the Barnes test in chapter five to see how well your thyroid is currently working.

DID YOU KNOW...

It is thought that as many as one in 50 people has a health problem resulting from an underactive thyroid. Recent research published in 2010 by the University of Exeter and the Peninsula Medical School in the United States has linked a chemical found in non-stick pans and water-resistant fabrics to an under-functioning thyroid. The researchers found that higher concentrations of the compound perfluorooctanoic acid (PFOA) in the blood correlate to a doubling in the rates of thyroid disease. PFOA is a very stable man-made chemical used to repel heat, water, grease and stains. It is used in the process of making common household and industrial items, including non-stick pots and pans, flame-resistant and waterproof clothing, carpets, sofas and curtains.

BINGO WINGS
The dangling fat hanging from your upper arms

BINGO WINGS ♀

If you have an excessive amount of fat on your triceps (the backs of your upper arms), commonly known as bingo, or bat, wings, you may have low levels of the hormone **TESTOSTERONE**. This powerful hormone, which is produced by both sexes (women produce much smaller amounts), promotes characteristics such as stronger, leaner muscles and reduced body fat stores.

Unfortunately, testosterone levels are falling in both men and women due to the effects of stress on testosterone production and a poor diet low in vitamins and minerals and essential fatty acids. Stress lowers testosterone hormone levels when the body uses pregnenolone (the base material it uses to make other hormones) to make cortisol, the main stress hormone, instead of making testosterone. High levels of cortisol therefore decrease the amount of testosterone available in the body. In women, this often results in bingo wings. I have seen high-powered, stressed-out female executives lose centimetres from their arms after starting my fat spot reduction programme, which gently boosts androgen (testosterone) production in the body.

DID YOU KNOW…

Low testosterone levels can impact negatively on health. Research suggests women with lower levels of testosterone are more prone to heart disease. A study of post-menopausal women published in 2003 in the *European Journal of Endocrinology* found that women who had atherosclerosis (a thickening of the arteries) had significantly lower levels of testosterone compared with women who did not have the disease. Studies also show that the treatments women take to control mid-life symptoms, such as HRT or low-dose birth control pills, can actually rob the body of testosterone. When these treatments are taken orally, they are broken down by the liver, which then produces a protein that binds to testosterone, causing a deficiency.

BIG THIGHS AND BUTT ♀

If you have an excessive and disproportionate amount of fat on your thighs and bottom, this tells me that you have a problem with excess **OESTROGEN** levels in your body.

Oestrogen is one of the main female hormones (although men do make some, too) that naturally promotes fat storage around the top of the legs and on the buttocks, and is a sign of female fertility when in proportion. The problem nowadays is that we are exposed to high levels of both natural and synthetic oestrogens in the environment. Synthetic oestrogen-like chemicals in everyday items such as plastic water bottles and non-stick coatings mimic the action of oestrogen in our bodies. The oestrogen-based contraceptive pill and hormone replacement therapy (HRT) are additional sources of excess oestrogen and also play a role in the creation of this fat spot. Do your legs chafe as you walk? Do you have problems finding jeans that fit? Then it's time to act to fix this fat spot.

BIG THIGHS AND BUTT

The large area of fat that makes it hard to exercise, and feels uncomfortable when you do so

DID YOU KNOW...

Drinking more than two cups of coffee daily can boost oestrogen levels in women, exacerbating this associated fat spot. A study conducted in 2001 found that women who consumed more than one cup of coffee a day had significantly higher levels of oestrogen. Women who consumed at least four or five cups of coffee had nearly 70 per cent more oestrogen during the early phase of their menstrual cycle than women consuming no more than one cup of coffee a day.

MOOBS ♂

MOOBS
Unsightly man boobs

MOOBS ♂

If you are a man and you have an excessive amount of fat on your chest (moobs), I expect you to have low **TESTOSTERONE** levels.

Testosterone promotes male characteristics such as stronger, leaner muscles, less fat and a deep voice. It also makes guys feel as though they are ten foot tall and bullet-proof. Unfortunately, as men get older they convert a percentage of what testosterone they are still making into oestrogen, the main female hormone that promotes fat deposition. Men can also produce oestrogen in their fat cells, which means that as men age and put on weight they produce more oestrogen, while their testosterone levels are already falling naturally.

So if your fat is turning you into a woman, it's time to do some testosterone-boosting exercise, eat better and work with me to restore a sense of male adventure to your life!

DID YOU KNOW…

I love this bit of research I unearthed: scientists have discovered that the excitement of driving a fast sports car makes the body produce more testosterone. The researchers recruited 39 young men to each drive a sports car for one hour. Saliva tests afterwards showed a marked increase in testosterone levels as the men drove around in the car, and researchers noted that the effect was most potent when the young male volunteers were driving through a town full of female admirers.

If you are a sports fan, you may be interested to hear that football teams that wear red might have an advantage over their opponents because the colour red can stimulate the production of testosterone.

Let me introduce **ALPHA 2 RECEPTORS**

Now that I have introduced you to the specific fat spots and my reasoning as to why some of us store excess fat in one or more fat spot areas, I hope you are beginning to understand how hormones can affect fat storage on the body. But there is one more known factor that influences how we can accumulate stubborn fat on our stomach, love handles and thighs and buttocks.

Hormones are not the only body chemicals that affect whether we lose or gain weight. I want to introduce you to 'receptors'. A receptor can be equated to a lock that a key (a hormone) fits into. Receptors and hormones work together to initiate changes and actions in your body. Interestingly, some receptors promote the breakdown of fat when activated by a hormone while others block the breakdown of fat.

THE ALPHA TRAP

Simply put, some fatty areas in the body have more receptors that block fat breakdown than receptors that increase fat breakdown. We are interested in 'alpha 2' receptors, as they are anti-lipolytic (in other words, they retard fat breakdown, which is not so good). Stubborn areas of fat have a high density of alpha 2 receptors, which makes it even harder for the body to break down fat in that area. And the fatter you are, the more alpha 2 receptors you have. This is known as an 'elevated alpha 2 trap'.

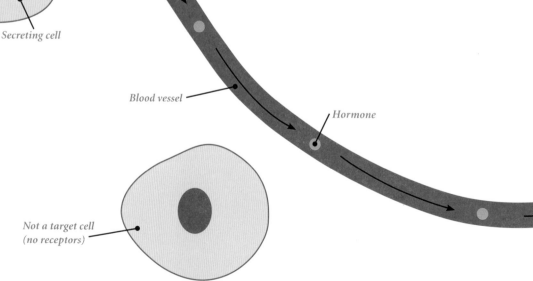

Secreting cell

Blood vessel

Hormone

Not a target cell (no receptors)

CIRCULATION IS VITAL

Touch the sides of your chest. Are they nice and warm? Now touch your buttocks, hips or thighs. Do they feel stone cold? This tells you that blood does not flow very well into fat deposits. This is important because it is the bloodstream that transports those hormones and natural chemicals that help to break down fat around the body. The flow of blood to fat deposits is also important because blood transports fat away from a fat cell to be burned elsewhere in the body.

THE SOLUTION

For those fat spots that are affected by the elevated alpha 2 trap, I recommend a particular exercise plan that promotes improved circulation and, in some cases, natural supplements for burning fat. So if your particular fat spot is your **STOMACH, LOVE HANDLES** or **THIGHS AND BUTTOCKS**, what you have to do is adhere to your particular fat spot programme with an intensity that would make a stalking lioness proud.

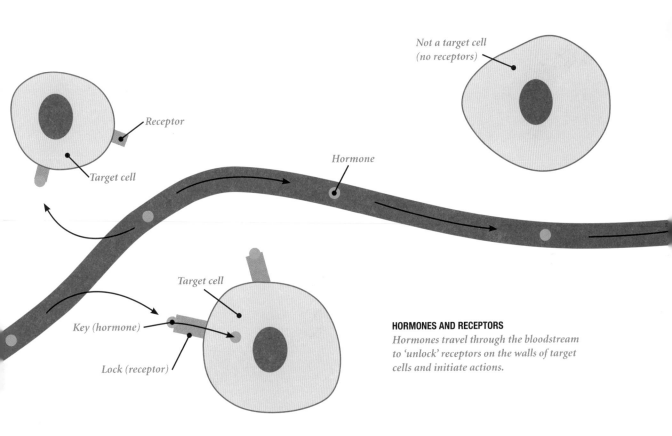

HORMONES AND RECEPTORS
Hormones travel through the bloodstream to 'unlock' receptors on the walls of target cells and initiate actions.

CHAPTER 2

A crash course in hormones

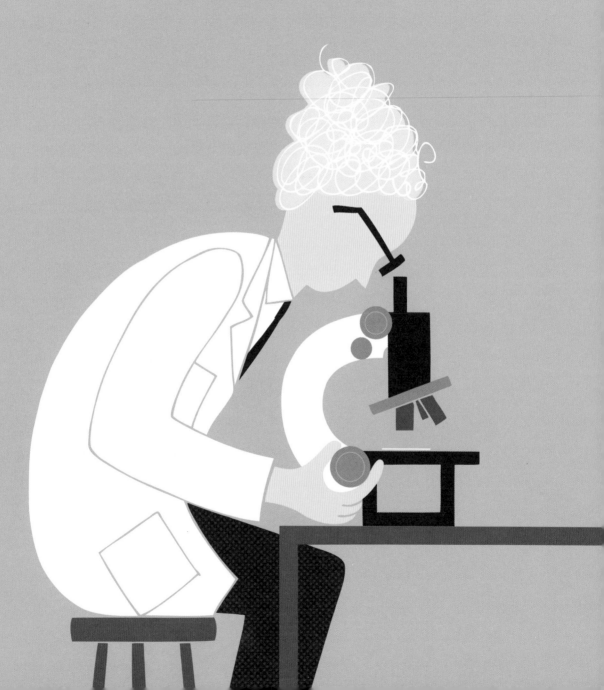

Hormones have a major influence on where and how you store fat. I have spent many, admittedly slightly boring, hours looking at scientific studies that prove this point. When I started my practice almost two decades ago the studies were scarce, but interest has picked up within the scientific community and I now have clear clinical proof that, for example, the hormones cortisol and insulin promote fat accumulation, and testosterone stimulates fat loss. Research on hormonal imbalances now shows clearly that disturbances in hormonal levels directly affect fat distribution. This chapter builds on this understanding, highlighting any hormonal imbalance you might have.

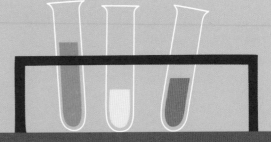

WHAT ARE HORMONES?

Hormones are essentially chemical messengers that are made in and sent from a group of glands and organs known collectively as the endocrine system. The endocrine system, along with the nervous system, controls and regulates all the internal workings of the body. The hormones produced by this group of endocrine sites influence and adjust a whole host of chemical and physical reactions in response to what is happening inside or outside the body.

In humans, the major endocrine glands are the hypothalamus, pituitary, pineal, thyroid, parathyroids, adrenals, islets of Langerhans (in the pancreas), ovaries and testes. Once the various hormones are released into the bloodstream from these specific glands and organs, they are sent to do essential jobs such as maintain normal blood glucose levels and control the menstrual cycle.

HOW DO HORMONES WORK?

Hormones transport vital signals from one cell to another. Most hormones act on cells by binding to a 'receptor' on the cell wall, or inside the cell. This is the lock (receptor) and key (hormone) scenario that I mentioned in chapter one (p20). The interaction of the hormone and receptor triggers changes within the cell that facilitate life, growth and immune function, and oversees reactions to stimuli such as cold weather or a tough exercise session. So hormones allow us to adapt, change and adjust according to our internal and external environment.

Hormone secretion is carefully regulated by the endocrine system so that just the right amount of a hormone is released into the blood to achieve a specific action. Incorrect amounts of a hormone can cause major problems in the body,

Blood vessel

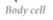
Body cell

Hormones

however. In children, for example, the human growth hormone (HGH) is designed to coordinate maturation and growth. Too much of this hormone and you may well have a giant on your hands; too little and a child's growth is stunted. Some hormones are released in short bursts, for example insulin, which is produced as your body digests a meal or snack. Other hormones are produced in a rhythm, such as progesterone in women, which helps to regulate the monthly female menstrual cycle. Keeping your hormones in balance and your hormonal system functioning optimally is one of the most important factors in maintaining your health, youthfulness, normal weight and body shape.

Take a moment to read this statement carefully. It is one of the most important facts in this book:

'Hormones exert a powerful influence on body fat distribution in humans'

I hope you now understand how important hormones are to life, health and a well-proportioned body. Our endocrine system strives to keep us alive, healthy and in balance at all times. The medical term for this is homoeostasis. Hormonal imbalances, on the other hand, may lead to weight gain in specific fat spot areas. I will explain how this can happen on the following pages.

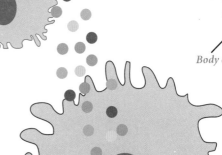

Blood vessel

HORMONE SECRETION
Hormones released into the bloodstream from different endocrine sites send signals from one point to another in the body.

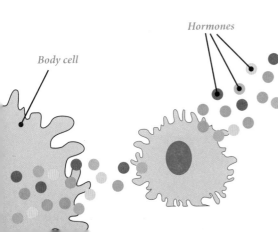

Hormones

Body cell

Body cell

INSULIN
...affects love handles ♀♂

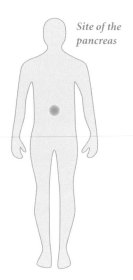

Site of the
pancreas

Insulin is produced in the pancreas and it moves glucose, the primary fuel our brains and bodies require to function, from the bloodstream into cells. Insulin is a powerful hormone and holds the key to delivering sufficient energy into each and every cell; without it, our cells would quite simply starve and die.

WHAT DOES INSULIN DO IN YOUR BODY?

The food we eat is converted into glucose, a simple sugar, through the process of digestion. The main sources of glucose are carbohydrates such as bread, rice and potatoes. The role of insulin is massively important: it is the only hormone that removes glucose from the bloodstream and delivers it into cells, where it is used as fuel. Any excess glucose that the cells don't require is diverted by insulin to be stored as glycogen in liver cells. When your blood glucose, or blood sugar, levels are low (I'm sure you know the feeling – shaky, irritable and slightly sweaty), the pancreas releases another hormone, glucagon, which does the opposite to insulin: it releases glycogen from storage in the liver to increase glucose levels in the bloodstream.

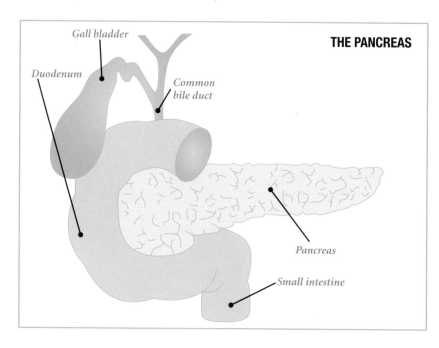

THE PANCREAS

Gall bladder

Duodenum

Common
bile duct

Pancreas

Small intestine

WHAT HAPPENS WHEN THIS HORMONE IS OUT OF BALANCE?

As we get older, our insulin levels rise and this may create problems and imbalances in the body, leading to big love handles, fat deposits on the linings of our arteries and diseases like stroke. In short, it is high insulin levels that may make you fat, accelerate your biological age and lead to a condition known as 'insulin resistance'. Insulin resistance occurs when the normal amount of insulin produced by the pancreas is unable to transfer glucose effectively from the bloodstream into the cells. The pancreas then produces more and more insulin in a vain attempt to get fuel into the cells. Unmanaged insulin resistance leads to a whole range of health problems such as abnormal blood lipids (cholesterol and triglycerides), high blood pressure and upper body obesity, all of which are risk factors for coronary heart disease (CHD). If left untreated, high insulin levels can progress to type 2 (adult-onset) diabetes.

HOW DOES BALANCING INSULIN HELP WITH WEIGHT LOSS?

The secret to reducing your love handles is to regulate and balance your insulin and blood glucose levels so they are neither too high nor too low. I have included cinnamon in your list of supplements (in chapter five) as a result of a recent piece of research published in May 2010 by the *Journal of Diabetes* (see resources, p157), which states that in human studies the spice was found to be very beneficial in cases of insulin resistance and weight loss.

DID YOU KNOW...

There is one other hormone that can influence blood glucose levels. Adrenaline, which is secreted in response to stress, stimulates the release of stored glycogen to provide a quick boost of glucose to meet the increased demand in energy required by the body to cope with the panic of a situation. This in turn makes the pancreas work harder temporarily to release enough insulin to cope with the excess glucose in the blood.

It is interesting to note that during periods of prolonged stress, however, production of the adrenal hormone cortisol increases and causes raised blood glucose levels (the hormone adrenaline gives you a quick burst of energy, but does not really impact on glucose levels, whereas one of cortisol's functions is to raise blood glucose levels sufficiently to enable the body to cope during the period of stress). The body then responds by producing more insulin to transport the glucose into the body's cells. Long-term stress levels mean that cortisol and insulin levels are constantly elevated, resulting eventually in insulin resistance. So now you know that stress can also make you fat and grow your love handles.

CORTISOL
...affects stomach fat ♀♂

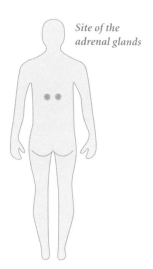

Site of the
adrenal glands

The adrenal glands sit on top of each of the kidneys and produce the hormones cortisol and adrenaline, which help us to deal with stress; without adrenal power we would not be able to rise to the occasion. We may complain of the stresses and strains of modern living, but we also tend to see stress as something that is fairly benign. However, it can have a very negative impact on your long-term health.

THE DIFFERENCE BETWEEN ADRENALINE AND CORTISOL

Adrenaline gives you a quick boost of energy and enables you to run from danger or turn around and fight. You experience a pounding in your chest, palpitations, cold sweats and butterflies in your stomach – all signs you notice first when you are feeling stressed. Other effects from the release of adrenaline into the bloodstream include: increased heart and breathing rate, which enables you to think quicker and gives you faster muscle response; blood is drawn away from the skin and clotting increases (in case you are injured and bleeding); blood is drawn away from your digestive tract to help reduce the possibility of vomiting.

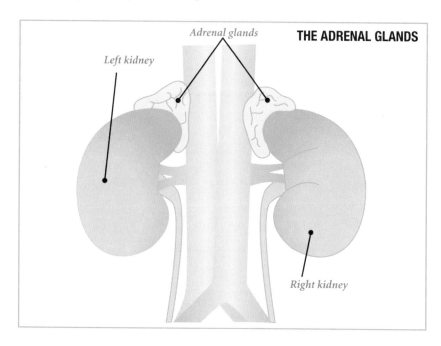

Adrenal glands

THE ADRENAL GLANDS

Left kidney

Right kidney

Cortisol, on the other hand, is designed to help you respond to long-term stress and stressors. It enables you to be on full alert for an extended period of time. Like adrenaline, cortisol also raises your heart rate, speeds your breathing up and drives blood to the muscles and the brain so you can act fast. But it also raises your blood pressure and increases the flow of glucose into the bloodstream to cope with the crisis and fuel the muscles in case you need to run away fast. This is really damaging in the long term, as sustained high blood glucose levels due to stress means high insulin levels (p27) and increased fat storage in the stomach area. Over time, high cortisol levels can cause accelerated biological ageing, abdominal fat deposition, loss of muscle and bone mass, heart disease and even damage to brain cells.

WHAT HAPPENS WHEN THIS HORMONE IS OUT OF BALANCE?

The human response to stress is all about action, alarm, energy and emergency. The body is designed to give a short, sharp, adrenaline-based reaction to the sudden appearance of a snake, for example. However, modern stresses don't end, as the kids need to be picked up every day from school, work deadlines keep getting tighter, the mortgage needs to be paid each month and the mother-in-law is not leaving. When faced with this long-term stress, the body moves into a phase governed by cortisol, or the 'resistance phase', as you hunker down for a long session of fighting and fleeing. This takes a big toll on the body as it tries to cope with the massive demands that stress places on it. Things can start to go wrong and you may experience erratic energy levels, high blood glucose levels, elevated cholesterol and poor sleep. The final phase is the 'exhaustion phase' and all that comes with it. You may find yourself waking in the early hours, retaining fluid, having dry skin, night sweats and high exhaustion levels. All this occurs while your stomach fat spot increases and your temper frays.

HOW DOES BALANCING CORTISOL HELP WITH WEIGHT LOSS?

Restoring cortisol to normal levels with the help of supplements can keep blood glucose levels stable and stomach fat to a minimum. Vitamin B5 and pantothenic acid, for example, have a marked therapeutic action on the adrenals, according to research published in 1983 in the *International Journal of Vitamin and Nutrition Research*.

DID YOU KNOW...

DHEA (dehydroepiandrosterone) is the most abundant hormone made in the adrenal glands. DHEA levels peak at around 22 years of age and then decline as we grow older. The reason why I mention it here is that improving DHEA levels helps to decrease overall body fat, especially in men. So as part of the action plan to overcome your stomach fat, we will tackle how to optimise adrenal function.

T4 AND T3
...affects bra bulge fat ♀

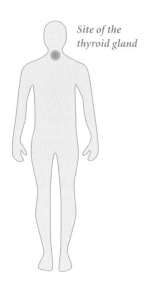

Site of the
thyroid gland

The thyroid gland is situated in the neck and controls the speed at which the body's chemical functions happen (metabolism) by secreting the hormones thyroxine (T4) and triiodothyronine (T3). These hormones also control how quickly the body burns calories and uses energy. If the thyroid releases too many hormones, you end up with hyperthyroidism: very thin and acting as though you have had 20 coffees before lunch. Too few of these hormones (hypothyroidism) and you burn fewer calories and pile on the weight.

WHAT DO THYROID HORMONES DO IN YOUR BODY?

Production of T4 occurs in response to a thyroid-stimulating hormone (TSH), which is produced in the pituitary gland. Much of T4 attaches to proteins in the bloodstream and is inactive. A tiny amount remains 'free' and this free T4 is converted into additional T3 in the liver and kidneys. As with T4, most T3 is bound to blood proteins, making it inactive, while the remainder is the biologically active form called free T3.

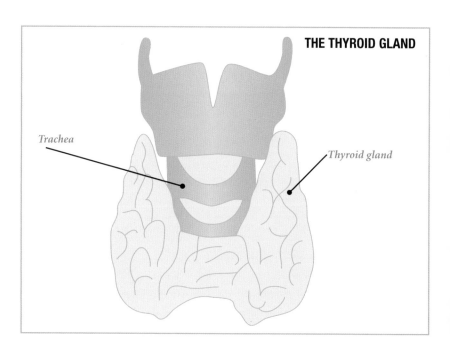

THE THYROID GLAND

Trachea

Thyroid gland

WHAT HAPPENS WHEN THESE HORMONES ARE OUT OF BALANCE?

The major signs of a sluggish thyroid function are fatigue, muscle weakness, dry skin and an inability to tolerate cold. People with this thyroid imbalance tend to fall into one of the two following categories:

★ An under-functioning pituitary gland doesn't produce sufficient quantities of the thyroid-stimulating hormone (TSH) so the thyroid fails to produce enough T4 (thyroxine).

★ T4 is not converted efficiently into T3.

A growing number of my clients have an autoimmune condition whereby they produce thyroid antibodies that attack their own thyroid gland. Unfortunately, thyroid autoimmune problems can go largely undiagnosed, as a routine thyroid test often doesn't pick up this problem.

There is another aspect to diagnosing a thyroid problem. 'Sub-clinical hypothyroidism' is a situation in which standard medical testing may not pick up a problem with your thyroid or your thyroid hormone levels, even though you have classic hypothyroid symptoms. This is frustrating, as you know there is a problem. This is where functional medicine testing (p10) steps in to provide an answer, as it looks very closely at minor changes in thyroid hormones and can pick up a slight dysfunction very early. My questionnaire in chapter three will help you to detect a potential problem in place of functional medicine testing, as will completing the Barnes test in chapter five.

HOW DOES OPTIMISING THYROID HORMONES HELP WITH WEIGHT LOSS?

It is the free form of T3 that increases your metabolic rate, heat production and the burning of calories. T3 also stimulates the breakdown of fats and helps to control two other hormones, cortisol and insulin, which promote fat storage. I have included the herb guggul (*Commiphora mukul*) in the supplements I recommend for this fat spot, as it has been shown to support effective thyroid function, especially through the increased conversion of T4 to T3 in the liver (see resources, p157).

DID YOU KNOW…

It is estimated that ten per cent of the UK and US populations have some form of hypothyroidism, and one out of every 4,000 babies is born with hypothyroidism. As many as ten per cent of women have some degree of thyroid hormone deficiency.

An additional concern with regard to thyroid function is the fact that during prolonged periods of stress, production of the adrenal hormone cortisol increases and this in turn creates a decrease in TSH production, which can also result in a thyroid imbalance.

TESTOSTERONE
...affects bingo wings ♀

Testosterone is not exclusively a male hormone. Women also produce small amounts of it in their adrenal glands and ovaries (on average, men produce between 4 and 10mg of the hormone per day, and overall have about 20 times more testosterone in their bodies than women). A woman in her 40s typically has roughly half the testosterone levels she had in her 20s.

WHAT DOES TESTOSTERONE DO IN YOUR BODY?

The exact role of testosterone in women is still unclear, but scientists believe it helps to maintain muscle and bone strength, is vital for brain function and contributes to sex drive, or libido. The idea that low testosterone levels contribute to fat accumulation on the backs of the upper arms arises from my conclusions that men do not generally have bingo wings. To me, the logical reason is that the higher testosterone levels in men help to create lean triceps. This assumption has been proved in my clinics as I work with female clients who have bingo wings.

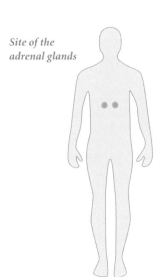

Site of the adrenal glands

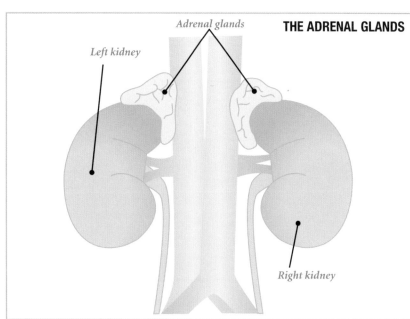

Adrenal glands

THE ADRENAL GLANDS

Left kidney

Right kidney

WHAT HAPPENS WHEN THIS HORMONE IS OUT OF BALANCE?

After the menopause or a hysterectomy (ovary removal), testosterone production in women may drop dramatically. Women with low testosterone levels may experience symptoms such as fatigue and low sex drive, and may find it very difficult to lose excess weight. HRT (hormone replacement therapy), which is prescribed to alleviate menopausal symptoms, may exacerbate the hormonal imbalance in some peri-menopausal women, exacerbating some symptoms and creating others. I believe it is vital that women who have the menopause are given a full hormonal test – one that includes testing testosterone levels as well as that of oestrogen and progesterone – to see which hormones they actually lack before being given HRT. A 'one size fits all' approach does not work with female hormones.

HOW DOES TESTOSTERONE HELP WITH WEIGHT LOSS?

Normalising or boosting testosterone levels in women will help to restore shape to the arms. It also improves bone density, mental acuity and increases libido. The targeted exercise programme in chapter five will also help to stimulate testosterone production.

DID YOU KNOW...

Symptoms of low testosterone levels in women may include: fatigue, definite loss of muscle strength and mass, weight gain, depression, increased risk of osteoporosis and related bone deterioration, increased risk of cardiovascular disease, vaginal dryness, lack of interest in sexual activity, painful sexual intercourse, sudden absence of menstruation, hot flushes and anorgasmia, or the inability to have orgasms.

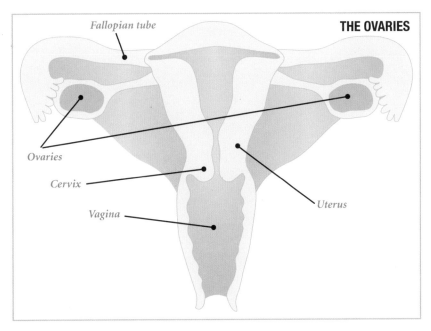

THE OVARIES

Fallopian tube

Ovaries

Cervix

Vagina

Uterus

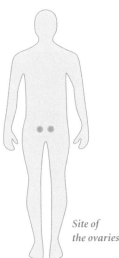

Site of
the ovaries

OESTROGEN
...affects the thighs and butt ♀

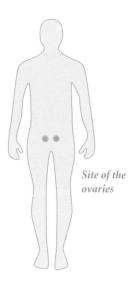

Site of the ovaries

The main female hormones are oestrogen and progesterone. Both men and women produce oestrogen, although the fairer sex makes a whole lot more of it. In women, oestrogen and progesterone work together to nourish and regulate the female sexual organs and breasts. These hormones also work in concert to ready the body for pregnancy and carry a baby to term. Oestrogen is produced mainly in the ovaries, but also in small amounts in the breasts, adrenal glands and in stored body fat. Progesterone is secreted by the ovaries during the last two weeks of the menstrual cycle.

WHAT DOES OESTROGEN DO IN YOUR BODY?

Oestrogen is largely responsible for female characteristics such as breasts and the development of the womb. It stimulates the growth of an egg within a follicle and plays a critical role in fertility and pregnancy. Oestrogen also reduces muscle mass, helps to retain calcium in the bones and – significant in the context of this book – promotes fat deposits on the bottom and thighs.

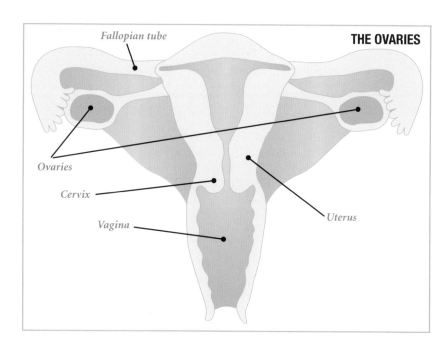

Fallopian tube

THE OVARIES

Ovaries

Cervix

Vagina

Uterus

WHAT HAPPENS WHEN THIS HORMONE IS OUT OF BALANCE?

Too much oestrogen may promote more fat deposition on the buttocks and upper legs, encouraging the classic pear shape that so many women dislike. An imbalance between oestrogen and progesterone levels may also create the uncomfortable symptoms associated with premenstrual stress (PMS) in younger women and menopause in older women. The majority of menstrual problems such as painful periods may also be due to excess oestrogen.

Oestrogen levels drop as a woman approaches the menopause. When she stops ovulating she stops producing progesterone and is classified as peri-menopausal. However, she may still be producing oestrogen. HRT (hormone replacement therapy), which is prescribed to alleviate menopausal symptoms, most often replaces both hormones and this may exacerbate the imbalance of oestrogen in peri-menopausal women, creating other symptoms. I believe that it is vital that women nearing the menopause are tested first to see which hormones they lack before being given HRT.

HOW DOES BALANCING OESTROGEN HELP WITH WEIGHT LOSS?

The excess of oestrogen that exacerbates fat storage on the lower half of the body can be corrected with the help of the herb *Vitex agnus castus*, as it is well documented (see resources, p157) as an effective treatment for hormonal imbalance, promoting harmony between oestrogen and progesterone. It is also used by herbalists to increase progesterone levels. This in turn helps to reduce fat deposition on the buttocks and thighs.

TESTOSTERONE
...affects moobs ♂

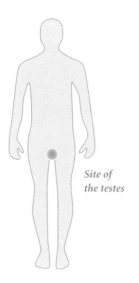

*Site of
the testes*

When you think of testosterone, what comes to mind? Macho men? Aggressive, impatient, alpha male attitude? Road rage? Violence? Testosterone's role in behaving badly is only part of the story. The hormone plays other important roles in health and disease that may surprise you.

WHAT DOES TESTOSTERONE DO IN YOUR BODY?

In men, testosterone is produced in the testes and is responsible for all the manly features – deep voice, facial hair, big muscles, lower body fat, sex drive or libido, lots of sperm and baldness.

WHAT HAPPENS WHEN THIS HORMONE IS OUT OF BALANCE?

As many men age, they find it harder to stay lean or lose weight. This is because by the time a man reaches the age of 50 his testosterone levels can have reduced by as much as 50 per cent of what they were in his potent youth. To make matters worse, as testosterone levels decline oestrogen levels may

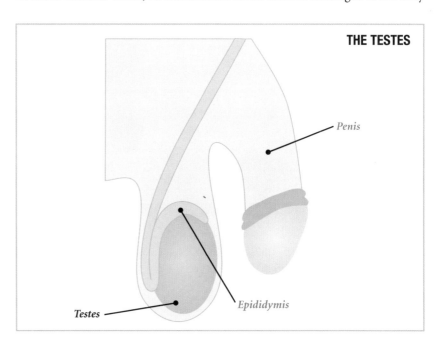

THE TESTES

Penis

Epididymis

Testes

increase: as a man's stomach grows fatter, the fat cells in the stomach produce the hormone oestrogen. (The possibility of young men having moobs tends to only occur if they are excessively overweight. This, again, is as a result of the fat cells producing oestrogen.)

The drop in testosterone levels as men age has been labelled by some experts as the 'male menopause'. Symptoms include a loss of interest in sex (decreased libido), depression, fatigue and moobs.

Stress also has a negative impact on the male body, as the adrenals produce high levels of cortisol in response to stressors and this, too, has a negative effect on testosterone levels.

HOW DOES TESTOSTERONE HELP WITH WEIGHT LOSS?

Normalising, or boosting, testosterone levels will help to restore muscle strength and develop healthy, defined and lean muscles. It should also improve bone density, mental acuity and increase libido. Simply follow the diet, exercise and supplement rules in chapter five and we will work together to restore your testosterone levels.

DID YOU KNOW...

Low levels of testosterone may increase the long-term risk of death in men over 50 years old, according to researchers with the Department of Family and Preventative Medicine at the University of California, Los Angeles, in the United States. Men with low testosterone levels were found to have a larger waist circumference, along with a cluster of cardiovascular and diabetes risk factors related to this type of fat accumulation. Men with low testosterone levels are also three times more likely to have metabolic syndrome (similar to insulin resistance) than men who have higher testosterone levels.

DID YOU KNOW...

Muscular young men are likely to have more sex partners than their less-fit peers according to David Frederick, a researcher at the University of California in the United States. He published a study in the *Personality and Social Psychology Bulletin* in 2007 suggesting that earning potential and commitment had less influence with women than virility and a muscular body.

CHAPTER 3

Analyse your fat

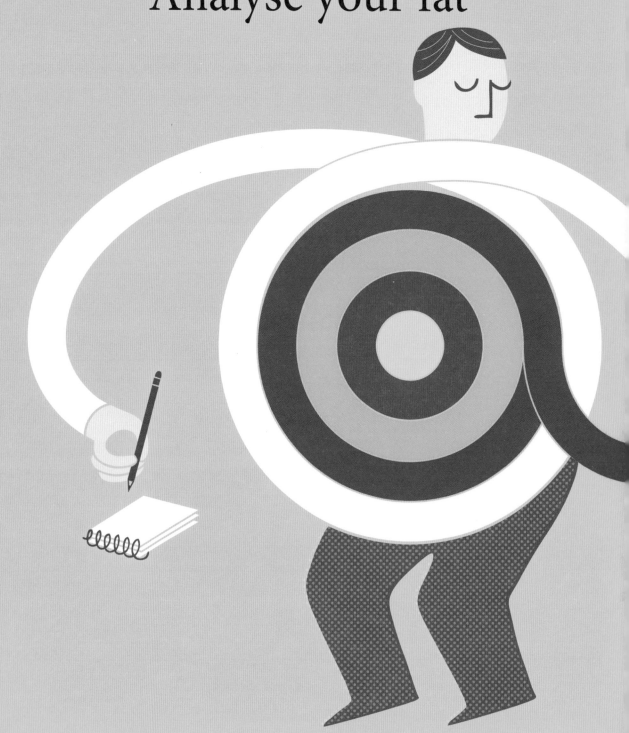

I have devised three different tests to help you quickly determine if you have a fat spot, and how urgent it is to tackle this problem. You may find that you have more than one fat spot; don't let this stress you, as the three tests will also guide you, helping you to decide which area needs your attention first. Be as honest as you can when you undertake these simple tests – they are not about punishing yourself, or letting yourself off the hook. Just stay calm and do them with an open honesty. It is now time for change, and change occurs when you face your fat!

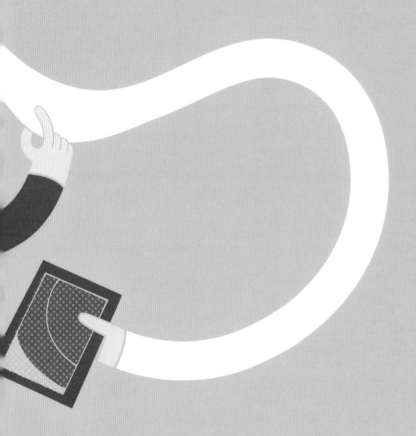

Establishing if you have a **FAT SPOT**

I believe that success with fat spot reduction starts with accurate planning and a good understanding of what you are facing. In my clinic I use specific functional medicine laboratory tests (p10) in addition to a thorough case history and visual check to determine if a client has a fat spot, but I have devised a special three-step process to enable you to analyse your own body instead.

1 I will ask you to take a long, careful look in the mirror at your body, visually pinpointing the fat spot, or spots, that need your attention.

2 You will then do a simple pinch test to confirm that the fat spot you have identified does indeed contain excess fat.

3 The last stage of the analysis is for you to complete a simple questionnaire on each of the fat spots that may be relevant to you. These questionnaires are a simple yet effective replacement for the functional medicine lab test results that I use in clinic.

A NORMAL BODY

It helps to see what a normal lean, healthy body should look like, as we don't often see normal bodies any more. There is no such thing as a perfect body, but notice the good proportions displayed in these two diagrams of a man and woman (opposite), which have no obvious accumulation of fat or fluid. In both cases, the torso is lean and the ribs are lightly covered by a small layer of insulating fat. The buttocks (not shown) are pert and heart-shaped. The insides of the thighs do not touch and the arms are shapely and lean.

Study the image that is relevant to you now. How far do you think your own body differs from this diagram?

Try to be as honest as possible about how you differ from the normal healthy male or female body depicted here, but don't be too critical of your own body. If you feel sad about the way your body currently looks and feels, let this negative emotion go, as it will prevent you from taking effective action. Accept that you have let things slip and concentrate instead on being determined to make amends and start caring for yourself so that you can bring your body back into proportion.

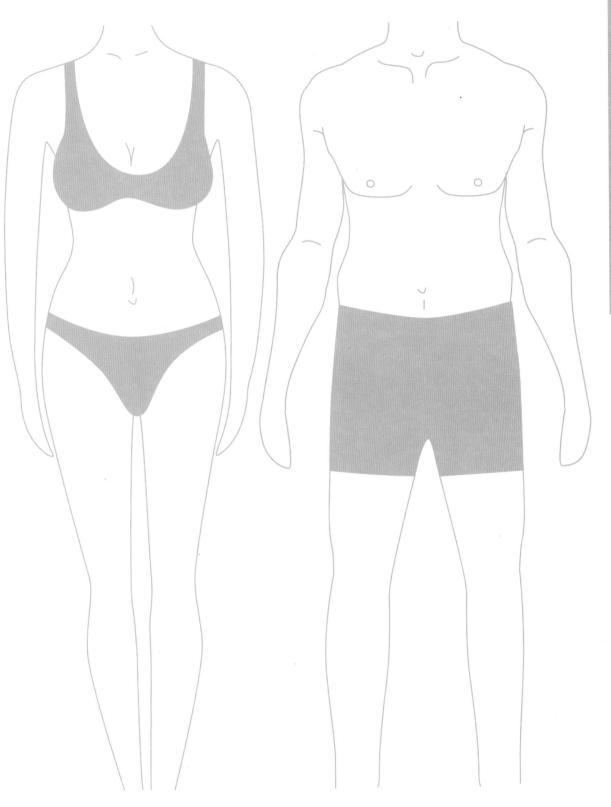

TEST 1 Rate your body visually

It is now time to face your fat spots. I am almost certain that you already know your problem area (or areas), but it is important that you stand in front of a mirror and look carefully, critically and yet lovingly at your own body.

1 Before you start, check that you have a full-length mirror, a hand mirror, a pencil and a camera to hand. No mirror? Buy one! Rating your body visually is an important part of assessing your body honestly and without prejudice so that you can move on and successfully tackle your current weight issues.

2 Now, stand in front of the mirror in your underwear. This is not about how much you hate your shape, but rather a process of deciding what areas need sorting out first. Can you see your problem area, or areas? Have a good, all-round look and take in your body shape. Can't see behind? Use the hand mirror and stand with your back to the full-length mirror to see the reflection of your bottom and back clearly.

3 The next step is to give different parts of your body a visual rating. Rate the potential fat spot areas – love handles, stomach, bra fat (women only), bingo wings (women only), thighs and bottom (women only) and moobs (men only) – on a scale of 1 to 5:

1 is perfect, svelte and 'glossy magazine' immaculate
5 is 'Oh my goodness!'
GOT IT?

HELPFUL GUIDELINES

✔ Always keep your fat spot in context. If you have a huge tummy and rate it a deserved 5, well done on being honest. But if you also give your slightly overweight thighs a 5 because you hate the way they look, your scores are going to be way out and useless.

✔ Don't pick on yourself, just try and be honest and objective (you may want to check your scores with a level-headed friend or family member).

✔ **SET A GOLD STANDARD FOR THE PART OF YOUR BODY THAT YOU RATE AS NUMBER 1.** We will use this spot as a comparison for all the major fat storage spots. Which part of your body is a 1, that is, slim and not hanging out or bulging? Everyone has a personal best spot. For most people this is the biceps – the front of your upper arms – so I recommend you use this area. Let your arms hang at your sides and have a good look and feel of this area. Pinch and poke it and get a sense of just how much fat is stored under the skin. It may be quite fat and soft, but that is fine. This is your base from which you compare your other fat spot areas. 'My biceps are a 1 and so my butt must be a …?' If your upper arms are not a good example of a 1, then find somewhere else. What about your calves or waist?

Now grab the pencil and start rating your body visually. Note down your scores in each small box as you work your way around your body.

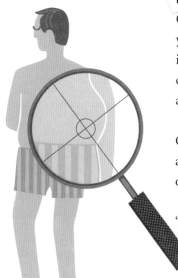

RATE YOUR LOVE HANDLES

Check out your love handles by grabbing the small hand mirror and turning your back on the full-length mirror. Have a good long look at your reflection in the small mirror. Do you see bulges of fat just above your hips that you can actually hold on to? You might even want to grab each love handle fondly and say goodbye.

Check out your baseline perfect spot (your biceps, if you have chosen them) and compare this against your love handles now. Then give yourself a rating of 1 to 5, please.

'My best spot is a number 1 so my love handles must be a number..?'

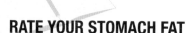

♂ [   ]   ♀ [   ]

RATE YOUR STOMACH FAT

Stand up straight in front of the full-length mirror, then turn to one side. Relax your stomach muscles completely, without stooping, and relax your shoulders. Then take a sideways look in the mirror at the shape of your stomach.

Don't suck it all in and cheat. You are done with cheating and just need to know the truth.

Now rate your stomach between 1 and 5. Remember, 1 is wonderful, 3 is starting to bulge noticeably, and 5 is just awful.

'My best spot is a number 1 so my stomach must be a number..?'

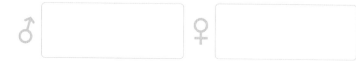

♂ [   ]   ♀ [   ]

RATE YOUR BRA BULGE FAT

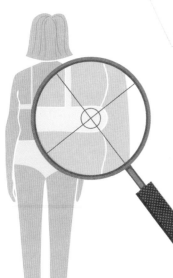

This is for women only. Stand in front of the full-length mirror, raise your arms slightly away from your body and analyse the area under your armpits. Is your bra nice and smooth against the sides of your chest wall or does it bulge with areas of fat trying to escape?

Rate your bra bulge fat now between 1 and 5.

'My best spot is a number 1 so my bra bulge fat must be a number..?'

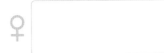

RATE YOUR BINGO WINGS

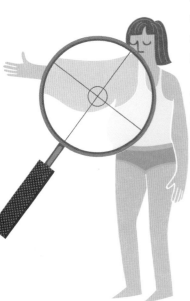

As you stand facing the full-length mirror, lift your arms away from your sides and hold them out at right angles to your body. Look at your upper arms. Do you have lots of loose flesh hanging down below your tricep muscles? Wobble your arms about a bit to be sure it's fat and not muscle (which shouldn't move).

Rate your wings now between 1 and 5. Think carefully before you put a number down. Try and see this area in context with the rest of your body.

'My best spot is a number 1 so my bingo wings must be a number..?'

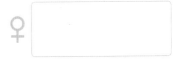

RATE YOUR THIGHS AND BUTT

The next part of your body that you need to take a good hard look at are your thighs. As you stand in front of the mirror, are your thighs rubbing together? Do you experience chafing?

Before you rate them, turn around, grab the hand mirror, and check out your bottom. Like what you see? Thighs and butts come in pairs and we need to tackle them together.

Now rate your thighs and bottom between 1 and 5. A quick reminder: if you have small thighs and a pert bottom, but lots of cellulite, you still need to be objective – we are not looking at cellulite. Judge your backside only on how fat it is, please. One is wonderful, and 5 is just not show business.

"My best spot is a number 1 so my thighs and bottom must be a number..?"

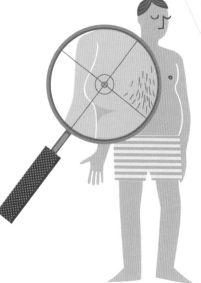

RATE YOUR MOOBS

OK, ladies, stand aside. Guys, stand up straight in front of your full-length mirror. Turn to one side without stooping or relaxing your shoulders. Then take a sideways look in the mirror.

Need a trainer bra? Be honest and rate your moobs now. Don't forget to rate your stomach while you are at it.

"My best spot is a number 1 so my moobs must be a number..?"

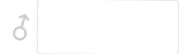

TEST 2 Perform simple pinch tests

You now need to test all your major body fat sites thoroughly and accurately using a simple skin-fold pinch test. The clear illustrations that follow show you exactly how to perform a skin-pinch analysis of your body fat. The results of the pinch test can then be combined in the table here with your visual observations to help you begin to form a clear picture of which area, or areas, need special attention.

To perform this test you will need a hard ruler or a rigid tape measure and a dose of patience. To get a feel for things, practice again on your biceps.

BODY PART	VISUAL SCORE	PINCH TEST
LOVE HANDLES		
STOMACH		
BRA FAT BULGE		
BINGO WINGS		
THIGHS AND BUTTOCKS		
MOOBS		

BICEP

Let one arm hang down at your side and keep the whole arm relaxed. Using the forefinger and thumb of your other hand, pinch a vertical fold of skin halfway between your shoulder and elbow, which should be directly over your bicep (the front of your upper arm). You should be gently grasping the fold of skin and an underlying layer of fat between your forefinger and thumb.

Take your time. Feel how much fat is beneath the skin. Be careful to only pinch the skin and fat, not the underlying muscle. If you are sure that you are just holding fat and skin, go ahead and measure the distance between your thumb and forefinger. Note this down on a spare piece of paper. Now ask a friend or someone close to you to do a pinch test on your bicep. Don't tell them what you measured. How do the two readings compare? If they are wildly different perform your own test again until you are confident that you have mastered the correct technique. Then pinch-test your body in each relevant fat spot area and write your scores down.

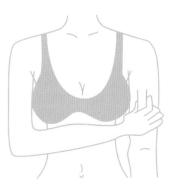

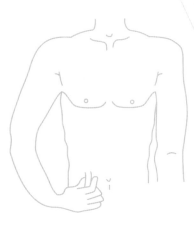

LOVE HANDLES

You may need help from a friend or a family member for this pinch test if you find it hard to twist your arm around to reach your back.

You should aim to lift a horizontal fold of skin and fat that sits directly over your kidneys, which are about five centimetres to the right and left of your spine. Locate the top of your hip bones first. From there, move your fingers towards the centre of your back and feel for your spine. Then feel for an area of fat at either side of it. Lift the fold of skin over your kidney with your right forefinger and thumb. Do this gently, as it can hurt.

Use your left hand – or ask your friend or family member – to measure the length of skin and fat as you pinch it away from your body.

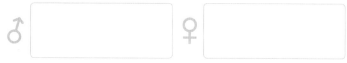

STOMACH

Stand up straight, pull your shoulders back and relax your stomach muscles. Pinch a vertical fold of skin and fat with your forefinger and thumb about two to three centimetres to the right of your navel (belly button). Make sure that you are pinching fat as well as skin (particularly if you have loose skin post-pregnancy).

If you are carrying a lot of weight here, you may find it hard to measure this area. Just do your best to get as accurate a measurement as possible.

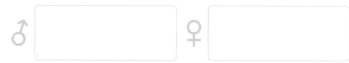

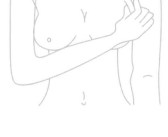

BRA FAT BULGE

Take your bra off for this measurement. Stand up straight with your shoulders pulled back. Using the forefinger and thumb of one hand, pinch a horizontal fold at the side of your chest directly below your armpit. Be gentle, as this is a sensitive area.

To double-check your measurement, perform the same pinch test on the other side of your body. The measurements should be the same, but if they are not, try measuring this area once more. Then note down the final result in the box below.

♀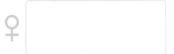

BINGO WINGS

Lift up one arm at right angles to your body and relax the muscles in your upper arm. Bring your other arm across your body and with your thumb and forefinger pinch a vertical fold of skin on the underside of the arm midway between the elbow and the shoulder. Remember to keep your arm relaxed as you do this. Then take the measurement.

If you want to double-check the measurement, perform the pinch test on your other arm.

♀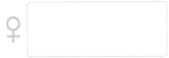

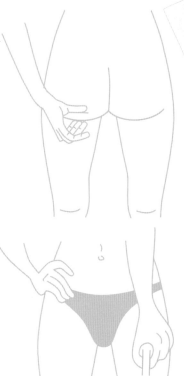

THIGHS AND BUTTOCKS

This pinch test is slightly more complicated, as you need to take two separate readings and work out the average.

1ST READING Keep your buttocks relaxed as you twist your upper body around slightly and reach down with a thumb and forefinger to pinch the area just above the crease that forms the boundary between the top of your leg and your buttock. Measure the fold of skin and note it down.

2ND READING Still standing, relax your thigh and pinch a vertical fold midway between your knee cap and the top of your thigh. Measure this fold of skin and note it down.

Add the two measurements together and divide them by two.

♀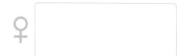

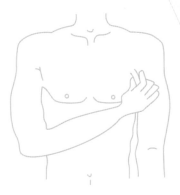

MOOBS

For this last pinch test, pinch a diagonal fold of skin and fat midway between your upper armpit and your nipple with your forefinger and thumb.

If you want to double-check your measurement, perform the same pinch test on the other side of your body.

♂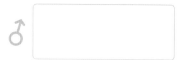

TEST 3 Complete the questionnaires

You have now had a good look and feel of your problem fat spot areas and rated them. Our eyes can deceive us though, so I have developed some questionnaires to take any guesswork out of your fat spot evaluation. I use these questionnaires in my clinic and they are an effective way to help you refine what you have already seen and felt.

Circle yes (Y) or no (N) to each question.

YES means that the issue is noticeable and is intruding on your lifestyle and your sense of wellbeing.

NO means that the issue is only occasional, or less than that.

If you can't decide the answer to a question, leave it and come back to it later. If you still can't decide, or you don't know the answer, leave it blank. When you have completed all the questionnaires, fill in the total numbers of 'yes's per question on the chart (the number of 'no's does not need to be recorded).

LOVE HANDLES

1. Do you struggle with your weight in spite of watching what you eat? **Y / N**
2. Have you experienced very high levels of stress over the past year or for long periods? **Y / N**
3. Do you suffer from poor memory or concentration and a 'fuzzy brain' after eating? **Y / N**
4. Do you regularly feel tired or lethargic, even after a good night's sleep? **Y / N**
5. Do you have high blood pressure (over 130/85)? **Y / N**
6. Do you have high cholesterol levels? **Y / N**
7. Do you get tired after a meal of at least 30 per cent carbohydrates? **Y / N**
8. Do you often feel agitated, jittery and moody? **Y / N**
9. Do you have polycystic ovaries? **Y / N**
10. Do you have skin tags – bits of skin that project from the surrounding skin anywhere on the body? **Y / N**

Total number of '**YES**'s for your love handles: _____

STOMACH

1. Do you wake often between 2am and 4am?	Y / N
2. Are you restless in your sleep?	Y / N
3. Do you sweat in your sleep?	Y / N
4. Do you have low blood pressure?	Y / N
5. Do you get shaky and irritable when you are hungry?	Y / N
6. Do you get angry suddenly?	Y / N
7. Have you experienced long periods of high stress?	Y / N
8. Do you overwork, with little play or relaxation time?	Y / N
9. Does your body hold onto fluids and do you look bloated?	Y / N
10. Do you suffer from indigestion and wind?	Y / N

Total number of '**YES**'s for your stomach: _____

BRA FAT BULGE

1. Is your axillary temperature below 35.8°C (96.4°F) for 8 out of 10 morning readings? (See p108 on how to perform this test.)	Y / N
2. Are you excessively tired and in need of lots of sleep?	Y / N
3. Do you suffer from constipation?	Y / N
4. Do you feel the cold much more than your friends?	Y / N
5. Have you had difficulty losing weight?	Y / N
6. Is your skin becoming dry and thick and does it feel cold?	Y / N
7. Has your period become heavier and longer?	Y / N
8. Is your hair beginning to thin and become dry and coarse?	Y / N
9. Are your nails flaking and splitting easily?	Y / N
10. Are your speech, movements and thoughts quite slow?	Y / N

Total number of '**YES**'s for your bra fat bulge: _____

BINGO WINGS

1. Do you have a diminished sense of wellbeing?   **Y / N**
2. Do you feel low and unmotivated?   **Y / N**
3. Do you suffer from persistent, unexplained fatigue?   **Y / N**
4. Is your libido low and do you have low sexual desire and pleasure?   **Y / N**
5. Do you have diagnosed osteoporosis?   **Y / N**
6. Have you noticed a decrease in muscular strength?   **Y / N**
7. Have you noticed changes in your ability to remember and think?   **Y / N**
8. Do you suffer from sleep disturbances?   **Y / N**
9. Have you noticed any body shape changes, especially on your arms and stomach?   **Y / N**
10. Are you menopausal and finding it difficult to lose excess weight?   **Y / N**

Total number of '**YES**'s for your bingo wings: _____

THIGHS AND BUTTOCKS

1. Are you on the mixed contraceptive pill or do you use the mirena coil?   **Y / N**
2. Do you suffer from premenstrual tension with nervous tension, weepiness, anxiety, mood swings and/or irritability?   **Y / N**
3. Do your periods start suddenly with heavy clots?   **Y / N**
4. Do you suffer from tender breasts or fibrocystic breasts?   **Y / N**
5. Do you suffer from vaginal dryness?   **Y / N**
6. Do you suffer menstrual cramps?   **Y / N**
7. Do you have problems with fertility and/or miscarriage?   **Y / N**
8. Do you suffer from fatigue and some depression?   **Y / N**
9. Do you have a low libido?   **Y / N**
10. Do you suffer from regular, cyclical headaches?   **Y / N**

Total number of '**YES**'s for your thighs and buttocks: _____

MOOBS

1. Do you suffer from flushes and sweats? **Y / N**
2. Do you suffer from a low sex drive? **Y / N**
3. Do you experience erectile dysfunction? **Y / N**
4. Do you suffer increased irritability and get cross easily? **Y / N**
5. Do you feel generally fatigued – have you lost your drive? **Y / N**
6. Do you have reduced muscle mass and strength? **Y / N**
7. Do you find it hard to concentrate? **Y / N**
8. Do you have decreased bone density, osteoporosis? **Y / N**
9. Do you do little or no exercise, especially with weights? **Y / N**
10. Are you gaining weight even though you eat carefully? **Y / N**

Total number of '**YES**'s for your moobs:_____

BODY PART	QUESTIONNAIRE SCORE	BODY PART	QUESTIONNAIRE SCORE
LOVE HANDLES		BINGO WINGS	
STOMACH		THIGHS AND BUTTOCKS	
BRA FAT BULGE		MOOBS	

Adding it all **UP**

Well done on completing the three different tests. Input your scores for each test into the final table on this page, add up the total scores and assess the results.

This example (right) of the final chart shows how the results of the three different tests should add up.

BODY PART	STOMACH
VISUAL SCORE	5
PINCH TEST	3cm
QUESTIONNAIRE	6 'yes's
TOTAL	14

BODY PART	LOVE HANDLES	STOMACH	BRA FAT BULGE	BINGO WINGS	THIGHS AND BOTTOM	MOOBS
VISUAL SCORE						
PINCH TEST						
QUESTIONNAIRE						
TOTAL						

FINAL TABLE

So what now? It's simple: if you have a pronounced fat spot, one that has a much higher score than the others, start by doing the detox plan and then follow the relevant fat spot programme in chapter five. If you have several pronounced fat spots, tackle your highest score first.

PHOTO TIME – THE CAMERA DOESN'T LIE

Before you get dressed again, take a photograph of yourself in your underwear. Make sure you include your fat spot.
Let it all hang out, please.

No one else needs to see this photograph. Refer to it when you get fed up with being on your six-week plan. Refer to it when you are craving a muffin and a piece of chocolate. Use the evidence on the photograph to motivate yourself to keep striving for your goal.

Look closely at your photograph. Happy with it? Enough said. You have your answer.

Time to act!

My fat spot

FOCUSING ON A POSITIVE OUTCOME

Having determined your fat spot, you need to feel primed and ready to go.

Think about why you want to reduce your fat spot. Don't reel off the same old reasons and responses. Be honest. This is the question you really need to answer. Get your reasons right, your purpose for losing weight right, and everything else will fall into place. True purpose attracts success.

Expect to achieve weight loss and reshape your body. Stop thinking negatively. Don't be scared to make mistakes as you tackle a new eating plan and exercise routine. If you want to achieve real weight loss and reshape your body, you need to believe you can achieve it and see the results change accordingly. Don't listen to anyone else. You have the tools and all the answers you need right here in this book. Take personal responsibility for your life, your weight, your shape and your decisions. Have faith in yourself. Be passionate and have a burning desire for success and you will make it. Commit to my plan in the following chapters and focus hard. You can change your weight **NOW**.

You also need to be persistent and disciplined. Be prepared to change your attitudes, beliefs and lifestyle. Expect to succeed. Those of my clients who don't achieve success act as if weight gain is something over which they have no control or power. They also don't set clear, realistic weight-loss and health goals, and then stop following the plan as soon as they hit an obstacle – a classic reaction that causes much weight-loss heartache.

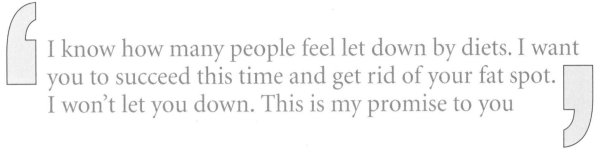

'I know how many people feel let down by diets. I want you to succeed this time and get rid of your fat spot. I won't let you down. This is my promise to you'

TOP TIPS FOR SUCCESS

★ My advice is to set clear, achievable goals and hold yourself accountable to the task and the time frame.

★ Follow the tailored exercise programme and my dietary and supplement guidelines that I have set out in chapter five and stick to them 100 per cent of the time for six weeks.

★ Change your mindset: consider obstacles an opportunity to learn to do something better or differently. Also ask for help from friends and family if you hit trouble.

★ Celebrate any loss of weight or change of shape by treating yourself to non food-based rewards. Go to the cinema to celebrate, for example.

★ Remember the positive health benefits of following this plan: you may experience lower blood pressure, improved heart health and lower cholesterol levels, decreased risk of developing diabetes, enhanced sex life, a better night's sleep, less aches and pains and a decreased risk of colon and breast cancer – a perfect vitality package.

★ Most important of all, if you follow my plan with no compromises or excuses, you will:

✔ restore your body
✔ optimise your health
✔ elevate your energy levels
✔ get back in proportion

CHAPTER 4

Prepare to attack your fat spot

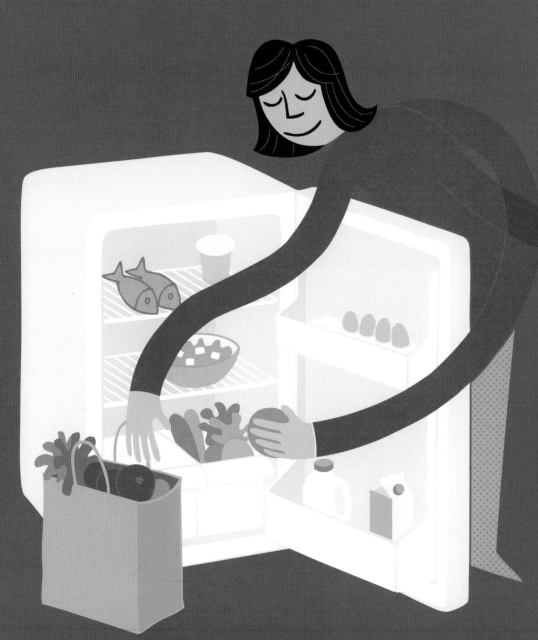

So much nonsense is written about cleansing the body that I am amazed anyone understands the concept of detox anymore. I recently read in a glossy magazine that a 'deep cleanse' weekend detox of eating maple syrup 'would leave you feeling energised and free of toxins'. Rubbish! For an effective detox – one where you reap all the health benefits – you need to do it properly. This is not an optional chapter, it is the first step in achieving targeted weight loss. So read on to find out how to gently coax your body into releasing years of accumulated junk from your tissues and fat storage areas.

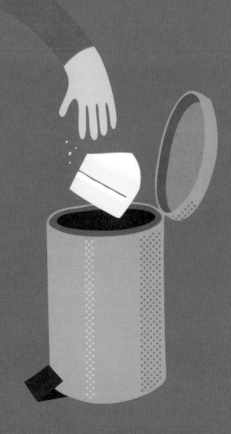

Why **DETOX?**

It's time for you to embark on a proper naturopathic detox as the preliminary stage in busting your fat spot, or spots. Proper detoxing is the basis of all successful treatments in natural medicine and is truly an amazing tool. I consider a naturopathic detox to be the ultimate preparation for a six-week fat spot plan.

I am often asked by my patients how long they should detox for prior to starting a fat spot programme. My advice is that the minimum time for an effective detox is seven days, which should help you get rid of some or most of the poisons you have stored away.

WHAT IS DETOXING?

You ingest a lot of poisons and toxic chemicals with the food (colourings, flavourings, pesticides, preservatives and so on) you eat and the liquids you drink, and you breathe in large quantities of toxins each day if the air you breathe is polluted. The breakdown and by-products of what you eat, drink and breathe need to be eliminated from your body.

   The liver, bowels (stools), skin, lungs and kidneys (urine) are all outlets for these poisons. The nervous system governs the elimination of toxins since it oversees all these organs, but if you are tired and stressed your nervous system will not govern this process as well as it should. This leaves your body unable to cope with the demands for elimination. If you are not eliminating these poisons, you are accumulating them: you start to store toxins in fat cells – your very own toxic dump. The more toxic you are the more fat you will need to accumulate to store the toxins, and the higher the chances are of your becoming ill. So the result is that you start putting on weight, holding onto fluid, changing shape and feeling unhealthy and below par. It is that simple.

THE SOLUTION

I take a very direct approach to the subject of targeted weight loss and ensuring that you will look your best. Everyone can be in great shape – you just have to have the correct advice and act on it. The first step in your bid to get rid of your fat spot is my seven-day detox plan based on solid naturopathic principles. You need to stop eating and drinking polluted foods and beverages and choose clean, detox-promoting foods instead. Buy organic wherever possible. This simple detox will leave you feeling energised and ready to attack your fat spot. As you embark on this two-stage programme of detoxing and then fat spot reduction, I will guide you through every aspect of regaining and maintaining your figure.

Detox plan – **THE RULES**

With simplicity in mind I propose a KIS (keep it simple) detox plan. I won't waste your time listing everything you can't eat and drink, instead I am going to concentrate on what you can eat and enjoy. Don't eat anything else!

✔ Breakfast on fresh eggs, fresh fruit and oat porridge.

✔ Lunch can be a colourful salad with cold-pressed extra virgin olive oil, fresh grilled fish and fresh asparagus. If you are vegetarian, add beans to the salad (kidney, haricot or similar).

✔ Dinner means a small green salad with a cold-pressed extra virgin olive oil and lemon juice dressing and a bowl of homemade vegetable soup with herbs and garlic added for flavour.

✔ Drink warm herbal teas, but no more than eight cups in a day.

✘ Resist all snacks except those on page 64.

✘ Avoid salt and all junk food.

✔ If you are hungry, either go for a walk or have a hot herbal tea.

✔ Buy a skin brush or loofah and give yourself an all-over exfoliation every day in the shower, as this helps to get rid of toxins. Make it a priority to buy the skin brush. For some reason many of my clients seem to forget to do this part – they pick and choose what to do and then wonder why they suffer adverse reactions to the detox.

✔ Rest as much as you can to give your nervous system the opportunity to get all the organs that eliminate toxins working at top speed.

✔ Your skin needs to breathe, as it is a pathway for toxins to escape, so let your skin soak up a little bit of sun if you are lucky enough to live somewhere sunny or it is summer. Five minutes of sun on each side of your body every day will also do your mental health the world of good.

SPECIAL NOTE OF CAUTION: If you are on medication, please ask your GP if it is alright to follow a healthy detox food plan for a week.

> 'Your KIS detox diet consists of a **low-saturated fat**, **mainly vegetarian**, oil-rich diet with **fresh fish** and **wholegrains**'

WHAT HAPPENS on a detox?

Expect to experience a variety of emotions and a few physical changes while you detox – after all, your body is undergoing a thorough cleansing process. Keep in mind that you are undoing what could potentially be years of slightly or very unhealthy habits. Letting go of bad habits can be quite a painful process, but remember that these habits are preventing you from being strong and healthy.

You will be hungry at times.

You will be a little tired and occasionally feel spacey.

You will be grumpy and short tempered at times.

You will feel sorry for yourself and want to eat chocolate.

You will be bored, especially if your usual focus is on food.

You will think about your favourite indulgence foods a lot.

You may have a headache for a few days and your nose may run as you eliminate toxins through your sinuses.

DAY 1 – You may be excited, but still apprehensive. Chill out! Shop for your food for the detox plan if you haven't already. Use the shopping list opposite.

DAY 2 – You will be feeling low, with a thumping caffeine-withdrawal headache if regular coffees through the day is your idea of heaven.

DAY 3 – You should be sleeping better. As the day wears on you may need a short rest, even a sleep.

DAY 4 – You should wake and feel refreshed, but try to rest today. This is crunch day. Stay focused even though you may want comfort food, hate detoxing and feel like crying.

DAY 5 – If you feel like raiding the fridge, go for a walk. Your tongue will be quite coated and your breath a little smelly by now. Brush and floss before going out. Your body is now officially detoxing!

DAY 6 – Ask yourself today if you really miss the alcohol, take-aways and chocolate. My bet is that you won't miss the way they left you feeling after eating them.

DAY 7 – At the end of today your detox is over and you can move on to start reducing your fat spot. Onwards and upwards.

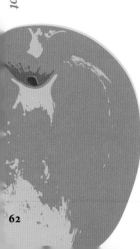

4

prepare to attack your fat spot

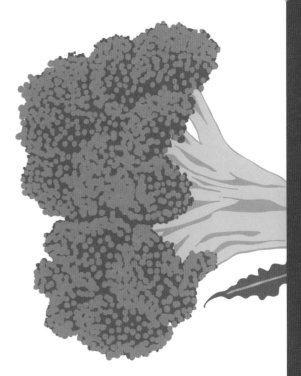

★ You should be able to continue working while you are on this detox plan, but be warned: you will be hungry. You may also want to organize your detox so that you complete days four and five over a weekend.

★ If you find it hard to sit down to eat a big lunch at a table with a knife and fork while at work, swap your lunch and evening meals around and take some soup in a thermos and a salad into work (see p66).

★ Rest and be peaceful. That means no parties, no after-work drinks, no family reunions and no late nights out.

FOODS TO BUY AND EAT:

VEGETABLES	FRUIT	SALAD	PROTEIN
Artichokes	All berries	Bean sprouts	Fresh fish
Asparagus	Apples	Cucumber	Organic eggs
Aubergines	Apricots	Mangetout	Tempeh
Broccoli	Fresh figs	Lettuce	Tofu
Butternut squash	Grapefruit	Onions	Organic smoked salmon
Carrots	Grapes	Tomatoes	
Cauliflower	Honeydew melon	Celery	**LEGUMES**
Courgettes	Mangoes	Chives	Chickpeas
Garlic	Nectarines		Green beans
Green beans	Oranges	**NUTS AND SEEDS**	Kidney beans
Mushrooms	Peaches	Almonds	Butter beans
Onions	Plums	Hazelnuts	Haricot beans
Peppers	Tangerines	Pecans	Pinto beans
Pumpkin	Watermelon	Walnuts	Pine nuts
Seaweed		Sunflower seeds	
Tomatoes		Pumpkin seeds	
		Sunflower seeds	

4

prepare to attack your fat spot

Suggested **MENU PLAN**

This is a detox menu, not a gourmet menu with foods and condiments to excite your palate and inspire you to new gastronomic heights. It is just simple, healthy life-enhancing food. If you remember this when you eat, you will cope well with the detox. Hundreds of my clients have been through it and succeeded; so can you.

Don't forget to:

✔ Eat smaller portions than usual

✔ Have a big glass of water as soon as you wake up

✔ Eat every meal from a plate at a table with a knife, fork and spoon so you feel as though you have eaten a proper meal. Chew your food well for optimum digestion

✔ Eat two pieces of fruit a day between meals if you are hungry – but no other snacks

✔ Rest if you feel faint

✔ If you feel really hungry in between meals and your energy levels are low, have some raw vegetable crudités or a bowl of warm vegetable soup

BREAKFAST IDEAS

Choose one of the following:

1 Egg/s (boiled, poached, scrambled) with steamed greens (eg, spinach) and smoked salmon pieces. Do not use butter or cream to scramble your eggs

2 Fresh seasonal fruit salad with a teaspoon of pine nuts or raw almonds

3 Wholegrain porridge (oats, spelt, millet, quinoa) soaked overnight in water and cooked with a little fresh apple juice. Serve hot with a few fresh berries

4 Detox juice

Detox juice recipe

5 carrots

4 stalks celery

4–5 spinach leaves

¼ head cabbage

3 sprigs dill, fresh

1 lemon with rind removed

Ensure that all the ingredients are rinsed or scrubbed, chop into smaller pieces if necessary, and juice. Pour into a glass and drink immediately.

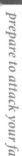

LUNCH IDEAS

You don't need anything fancy for lunch, just fresh, unprocessed foods. Don't add anything that is not included in the shopping list (p63).

Your meal should be divided into three portions:

1 ONE THIRD should be a well chopped raw salad. Make sure you include three different coloured vegetables. Wash the salad very well and drizzle over a dressing of lemon juice mixed with a little cold-pressed extra virgin olive oil. Chew the salad very well before you swallow, as it can be hard to digest and will give you wind if you don't.

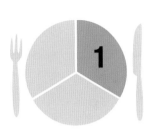

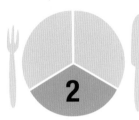

2 ONE THIRD should be steamed vegetables that still taste crunchy. (If you are at work and can't prepare steamed vegetables, feel free to have a huge salad that incorporates two portions.)

3 For the **LAST PORTION** choose one of the following:

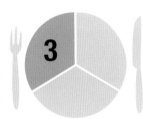

★ Vegetable soup. Soups are a fantastic lunch option – add some pulses and wholegrains to the recipe, but make sure you use mainly vegetables. For example, make a tomato soup (made from canned tomatoes) with some fresh basil and black-eyed beans added. Look online for good detox, stock-free soup recipes and avoid adding pepper and salt or any other condiments

★ Mixed vegetables and brown rice with tomato purée. Pre-cook the rice and ensure that the vegetables are still crunchy. Heat the tomato purée, mix into the rice and vegetables and serve piping hot. Try adding chillies and some fresh herbs to taste

★ Brown rice with stir-fried asparagus, onion, leek, spinach, black-eyed beans. Cook the rice first, then lightly stir-fry the vegetables in cold-pressed extra virgin olive oil before stirring in the rice and serving

★ Fresh grilled fish or smoked salmon

★ Grilled tofu or tempeh with baked onions and garlic cloves in their skin

★ Lentils cooked with garlic and onions and served with baked vegetables

★ Warm mixed bean salad with chopped vegetables and fresh herbs

NOTE Feel free to eat lots of fresh salad (1) and vegetables (2), but go easy on the last portion (3).

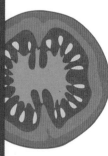

DINNER IDEAS

1 Start your meal with a small plate of chopped salad tossed in a dressing of lemon juice and cold-pressed extra virgin olive oil. You are free to design your own salad, but I love avocado, tomatoes, fresh basil, mixed leaves, grated cucumber and raw courgettes.

2 Have a bowl of fresh homemade soup.

I want you to take the time to cook fresh food. Part of the problem with most people's diets is that they want easy, quick food, which often justifies the reason for ready meals. This detox plan is about spending a little time getting your diet sorted and benefiting your body.

Take, for example, soup: all you need to do is cook a combination of vegetables that appeal to you and blend them in a food processor or blender. You may use chilli to taste to add extra bite and flavour if you like. If you make enough soup, you can refrigerate some for the next day and have a small mug of the soup again shortly before bedtime so that you go to sleep feeling full.

This is an example of a free soup recipe that you can find online. It took me 30 seconds to find and about 20 minutes to cook. It is my favourite find: a creamy spinach soup that contains no cream.

Spinach soup
(Makes enough for three portions)

2 tbsp cold-pressed olive oil	Heat the oil in a saucepan over a medium heat. Add
1 medium onion, diced	the onion and sauté for a few minutes until soft. Add
1 heaped tsp garlic, chopped	the garlic, carrot, celery and leek and sauté for two
1 medium carrot, diced	minutes. Pour in the water and add the bay leaves
1 celery stalk, diced	and thyme. Bring everything to the boil, reduce the
1 medium leek, diced	heat and simmer gently for 15 minutes or until the
1.4 litres water	vegetables are soft. Remove the pan from the heat and
2 bay leaves	remove the bay leaves and thyme. Purée the broth,
1 sprig of thyme	return it to the saucepan and add the spinach. Cook
1kg fresh spinach, chopped	over a medium heat for a few minutes until the spinach
	wilts. Serve hot and refrigerate the remaining portions
	for other meals.

prepare to attack your fat spot

HOW WELL DID YOU COPE WITH THE NATUROPATHIC DETOX?

One hundred per cent adherence? You get a gold star. You have what it takes to bust your fat spot. **WELL DONE**.

Some cheating, but nothing you are not prepared to admit? You just slip in under my radar, so read on.

Cheated quite a bit? I suggest that you **GO BACK TO THE START OF THE CHAPTER** and pretend that you have not just blown seven days. Start how you mean to go on. See you back here in seven Groundhog Days.

TAKE STOCK AND SET YOUR GOAL

Now that you have completed your detox, I want you to set a goal for the next six weeks. If you skip this process, you are setting yourself up for failure. If you don't know where you are going, how can you expect to get there? Aimless dieting is nonsensical. Ultimately it's you who has to undertake the plan, see the future and work towards your dream so make your goal personal and achievable: to complete the next six weeks with patience, diligence and total commitment, to get your body back in proportion and be pleased once again with your body shape. Write down your goal, put the piece of paper up on the fridge or your bathroom mirror and look at it every day. There is absolutely no point in setting a goal and then never looking at it again. Your fat spot goal needs to be in your face whenever you think about food.

PREPARE YOUR MIND, FRIENDS AND FAMILY

You are going to need help with this fat spot mission. If weight loss was easy, you would not be reading this book. So here are a couple of golden rules to help you survive.

RULE 1

Ignore input from anyone who is not slim, healthy and energised. If someone who is fat and tired gives you any dietary or lifestyle advice, especially about not doing 'a fat spot diet', ignore them or lend them a copy of this book.

RULE 2

Find someone you trust who loves you and wants you to be leaner and in proportion. Ask them to be your rock and your conscience as you progress through the programme.

CHAPTER 5

Time to take action

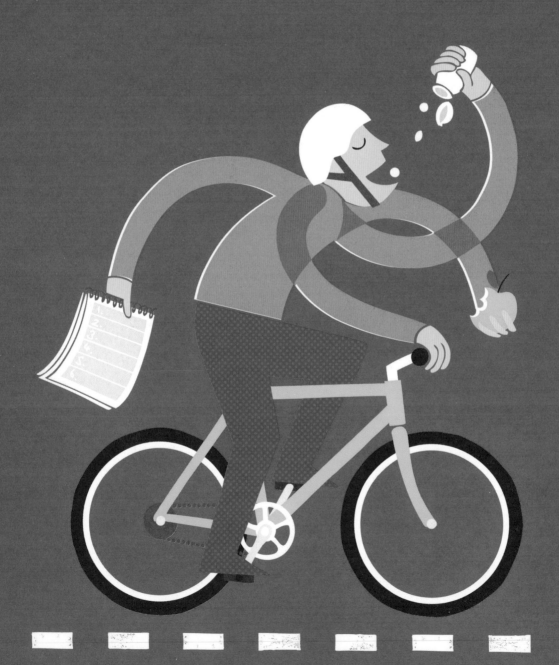

Now is the time to put your energy and effort into getting rid of your fat spot, or spots.

I have made my basic dietary plan (which is explained in detail at the beginning of this chapter) as simple as I can. There is nothing fancy about it; it is just a food plan that works. Please feel free to search out recipes from books and online information, but don't break my simple rules.

For each fat spot, I take you through a summary of the specific dietary, lifestyle and environmental factors that may be influencing the location of your stored fat. I also list the nutritional and herbal supplements that you will need to take to boost your fat loss. Skip the supplements at your peril! They work and are essential to your success.

Exercise is also vital if you want to see great results. There is some important information about how to exercise after my basic dietary plan, and then at the end of each fat spot section there is a professionally designed, tailor-made fat spot exercise programme for you to follow for the next six weeks. These inspiring, motivational programmes are neither difficult nor overwhelming, so embrace the challenge!

Max's **MEDITERRANEAN DIET**

My optimal food plan is based on the dietary principles that govern the way people typically eat in the Mediterranean region. Why? Because this is the healthiest way to eat in the long term. The basic principles of a Mediterranean diet are what I want you to follow for ALL the fat spot programmes EXCEPT moobs, although each fat spot also includes its own additional specific dietary recommendations.

A recent article in the *British Medical Journal* sums up why I want you to embrace a Mediterranean-style diet:

'Scientific studies have proven that the Mediterranean style of eating has a lowering effect on high blood fat levels (cholesterol and triglycerides), reduces insulin resistance and raises the levels of protective antioxidants such as lycopene (which is found in tomatoes)'

BASIC MEDITERRANEAN DIET (MD) PRINCIPLES

VEGETABLES AND FRUIT, LEGUMES AND BEANS, WHOLEGRAINS AND HEALTHY FATS — 50%

FRESH FISH — 25%

EGGS, POULTRY, CHEESE (GOAT, COW, SHEEP), NUTS AND SEEDS — 15%

LEAN MEATS — 10%

I have spent over 25 years looking at what people eat, and I am now convinced that the Mediterranean cuisine is the one dietary system I feel comfortable recommending as the basis for all healthy eating. I know the Mediterranean approach to eating well, as my lovely wife is Portuguese, so it is with a glad heart that I recommend it. It is time for you to stop eating calorie-dense, nutrient-depleted processed foods and enjoy the wonderful health benefits that a Mediterranean (MD) diet can bring.

The table (left) neatly sums up what a Mediterranean diet comprises. The majority of your daily intake of food should consist of vegetables and fruit, and you should also include some wholegrains and a little unsaturated fat. Before my clients embark on one of my programmes, they each complete a seven-day food and drink diary, carefully noting down what they eat each day. I am often astonished when I read the results. Over 68 per cent of my clients rarely eat fresh fruit, 38 per cent 'don't like or eat vegetables', and a staggering 67 per cent under the age of 40 choose to eat only potatoes and peas as their vegetable portions. Vegetables and fruit provide essential nutrients, and my rule with my clients is that if they miss one of their five portions of vegetables in a day, they should eat six portions the next day.

Fresh fish should also figure frequently in your diet. Include poultry and dairy produce occasionally, and eat red meat infrequently. I go into more detail with my **SIMPLE RULES** (p72), so read on to find out exactly what my optimal diet entails. If you can afford it, please try to buy organic produce whenever you can so that you eat good-quality chemical-free healthy food.

Don't forget that I will also highlight particular foods to eat and what to avoid within each fat spot programme in this chapter, and I will also give you ideas on how to put a menu plan together.

IMPORTANT NOTE

Most of my fat spot diets induce a further period of detox in addition to what you experienced during your week-long detox (chapter four), which is what happens when you stop eating unhealthy foods. For a few days you may feel as though you have the flu, with aches and pains, poor sleep patterns, general fatigue and a headache. This is normal; your body is taking the opportunity to do some more internal cleansing. Please persevere and don't use these symptoms as an excuse to bail out of my eating plan.

The sugars and processed foods listed below can produce harmfully high glucose levels and a high insulin response: when insulin levels are high, your body converts blood sugar into energy and stores extra energy as fat. In addition, a diet that consists mainly of high GI foods (pp96–97) can lead to carbohydrate cravings and an overall increase in appetite – potentially creating weight gain, fatigue and fluid retention. These foods can cause large fluctuations of both blood glucose and insulin levels, leading to a vicious cycle of overeating and fatigue, so avoid them.

★ Sweets
★ Sugar, all types
★ Honey
★ Sucrose
★ Alcohol
★ Biscuits and cakes
★ White potato
★ Chips and crisps
★ Sweetened cereals
★ Sweetened fizzy drinks
★ Sweet snacks
★ White bread
★ White pasta
★ White flour
★ White rice

SIMPLE RULES

I recommend 15 key requirements for my MD diet. Please implement these changes to your diet as soon as you can. None of them is particularly demanding, yet the cumulative benefits are huge:

1 DO NOT EAT SUGAR

Sugar elevates the amount of glucose in your blood very quickly, which in turn is stored as fat. Think of body fat as unwanted, unused sugar. Do not add sugar to any food or drink, and avoid sugary foods. That means no confectionery (sweets, cakes and biscuits) fizzy drinks, pancakes, ice cream – I could go on forever! If you are still not sure what to avoid, take a look at the box on high GI foods on page 97.

2 LOVE YOUR VEGETABLES

I expect you to eat five portions of vegetables every day from now on. Enjoy them lightly steamed, roasted, raw in salads or even boiled if you have to. Frozen vegetables are fine, and organic is best. One portion is approximately one medium-sized carrot or a handful of beans, for example.

3 HAVE A HIGH INTAKE OF FRUITS

Eat a minimum of two portions of fresh, organic, washed fruit every day, even in midwinter. Fruit is packed with fibre and natural chemicals that ignite good health in your body. Just remember that the fruit must be as fresh as possible for the maximum nutritional benefit; the older the fruit, the more impaired its nutrients. See the box (opposite) for guidelines on fruit portions.

4 HAVE A HIGH INTAKE OF LEGUMES AND BEANS

Not sure what a legume is? The list includes chickpeas (garbanzo), lentils, butter beans, soya beans, green beans, dried peas and black beans. They are all fabulous sources of fibre, protein and minerals, and should play a major part in your daily culinary experience. Add legumes and beans to soups, toss them into salads and search cookbooks for inspiration. I use lentils in place of white rice, especially when cooking fresh fish or grilling chicken.

5 HAVE A REGULAR INTAKE OF FISH AND SEAFOOD

Fish is eaten on a regular basis in the Mediterranean region. Oily fish such as mackerel, river trout, herring, sardines, albacore tuna and salmon are known to be rich sources of healthy omega 3 fatty acids. This wonderful fat protects your heart, improves your skin and generally perks your body up. There is a problem though: oily fish is also very polluted. Some of these fishes are contaminated with high levels of dangerous mercury and an even nastier chemical called polychlorinated biphenyls (PCBs). So my recommendation is that you eat oily fish once a week only (small oily fish such as mackerel and sardines are better than tuna) and eat white fish at least twice a week.

NOTE: Adding linseeds (also a fabulous source of fibre if added to muesli or salads) and organic linseed oil to your diet will also top up your omega 3 levels without the risk of ocean-based contaminants.

6 HAVE A REGULAR INTAKE OF A VARIETY OF WHOLEGRAIN CEREALS

Whole means everything, and in the case of grains it means eating a product that has its vitamins and fibre intact; you get the full health benefits from these foods, as nature intended. Please buy only wholewheat pasta, wholemeal or wholegrain bread and brown rice. Variety means that you need to break your wheat-based carbohydrate diet if you eat endless sandwiches and toast. There are some fabulous grains, including millet, quinoa, amaranth and rye, so start experimenting with them in recipes.

7 HAVE A VERY MODERATE INTAKE OF ALCOHOL

I think one glass of wine every day is fine, and I am persuaded that it may also have physical and emotional benefits. However, if you drink more than a glass a day, succumb to drinking binges or use alcohol to relax, you need to stop drinking or limit yourself to my drinking recommendations. My diet allows women to enjoy one small glass of wine (148ml) daily and men to drink no more than one medium glass of wine (296ml) a day.

8 HAVE A LOW INTAKE OF MEAT

Animal fat is an obvious risk factor for heart health. I want you to dramatically reduce your consumption of **RED MEAT**. You can, however, have organic chicken (take the fatty skin off first) and turkey twice a week. If you really cannot do without red meat, treat yourself to a piece of organic lean red meat once every three weeks. I can hear you cry, 'But how do I get my iron?' Leafy green vegetables are a very good, healthy source of iron and as you will be eating five portions of vegetables a day make sure you include plenty of spinach, Swiss chard, peas, asparagus, parsley, Brussels sprouts and beetroot.

WHAT IS ONE PORTION OF FRESH FRUIT?

★ Small-sized fruit:
One portion is two or more small fruits. For example, 2 plums, 2 satsumas, 2 kiwi fruit, 3 apricots, 6 lychees, 7 strawberries, 14 cherries

★ Medium-sized fruit:
One portion is one piece of fruit. For example, 1 apple, 1 banana, 1 pear, 1 orange, 1 nectarine

★ Large fruit:
One portion is, for example, ½ grapefruit, 1 slice of papaya, 1 slice of melon (5cm slice), 1 large slice of pineapple, 2 slices of mango (5cm slices)

5

time to take action

9 HEALTHY FATS, NOT NO FAT

My MD diet isn't designed to eliminate fat from your diet, but rather to make wise choices about the types of fat that you do eat. I strongly discourage you from eating foods high in saturated fat (specifically cows cheese, butter and fatty meats, which all contain animal fat) and hydrogenated oils (margarine), as they can contribute to heart disease. My rule of thumb is that if a fat goes white and hard at normal room temperature, it is probably going to do the same in your arteries. However, some fats – namely monounsaturated and polyunsaturated fats – in small quantities are good for you. Olive oil is an example of a monounsaturated fat, and cold-pressed extra virgin olive oil contains the highest levels of the protective plant chemicals that help you to stay healthy. I love organic olive oil; try adding a drizzle of it to all your salads and vegetables.

10 HAVE A LOW INTAKE OF COWS DAIRY PRODUCE

Drastically reduce your intake of full-fat hard yellow and soft white cheeses, as they are loaded with high-calorie fat. However, you can eat white sheep or goats cheese occasionally – my favourite is feta cheese, and halloumi and mozzarella are also fine (as is cottage cheese). You should also aim to have a daily portion of probiotic natural unsweetened yoghurt (if you don't have it for breakfast, add it to a bowl of soup or a dish of pasta, for example). The calcium in cows, sheep or goats yoghurt is important for bone health, and the friendly bacteria in live yoghurt will help to soothe your digestion and boost your immune function.

11 INCLUDE HERBS AND SPICES

Herbs and spices add flavour and aroma to foods and reduce the need for salt or fat when cooking. They are also rich in a range of health-promoting antioxidants. Experiment with fresh herbs such as coriander, basil and thyme and spices like turmeric, paprika and ginger.

12 EAT EGGS

The idea that eggs raise your cholesterol levels is now well and truly debunked, so enjoy better health by eating more eggs. Eggs are a good source of high-quality protein, and a very useful ingredient or basis for a meal. I always eat organic eggs, which adds about one pound to my weekly shop – not a lot to pay for a healthier egg.

13 ENJOY NUTS AND SEEDS

Keep packs of raw organic almonds, cashews, pistachios and walnuts to hand and have a small palmful as a quick snack. Don't overdo nuts, though, as they are calorie-dense. The same rules apply to seeds. They are packed with goodness, but are also high in calories. Try adding a couple of teaspoons of mixed sesame and sunflower seeds to your salads.

14 CHECK YOUR PORTION SIZE

Foods at the top of the MD table (p70) can be eaten and enjoyed in larger amounts and more frequently, but your portion sizes and frequency of eating should decrease accordingly in the lower sections.

15 ENJOY COMPANY AT MEALTIMES

Food should create enjoyment and pleasure, so eat your meals in the company of others if possible, and savour each mouthful.

TAKING GENERAL NUTRITIONAL SUPPLEMENTS

I believe that you can't and don't get enough vital nutrients from food: essential, life-promoting nutrients are often missing from modern foods (intensive farming methods, soil depletion, food processing, poor cooking methods and excessive food miles rob food of much of its natural goodness). Environmental pollution and our hectic lifestyles also mean that we have an ever-increasing need for nutrients that will protect us and allow us to function effectively.

I recommend that you take two general supplements every day in addition to adhering to my MD diet. A multivitamin and mineral supplies many basic nutrients that the body requires to regulate the production and breakdown of hormones. You also need to supplement your diet with omega 3 oil capsules. Ask at your local store for a high quality fish oil product (see box, right) so you don't ingest polluted fish oils.

HOW TO BUY, WHAT TO LOOK FOR

Buy good-quality nutritional supplements from a reputable health food store or a health professional such as a naturopath or nutritionist. Health food store staff are usually very knowledgeable about good-quality products and are keen to help. If they aren't, shop elsewhere. I don't recommend buying supplements from a pharmacy, as the staff are often not as knowledgeable. It is also fine to buy supplements online from a reputable site, but keep in mind that you get what you pay for. Cheap supplements mean one of two things: low active ingredient levels or a scam. Quality raw materials cost money, as does correct pharmaceutical grade manufacturing. So shop wisely and always ask questions before you buy.

There is more detailed information on daily multivitamin and mineral and pure fish oil supplements in each fat spot section within this chapter.

FISH OIL SUPPLEMENTS

These are the requirements that must be met by a fish oil supplement before you purchase it:

★ Undetectable levels of the heavy metal mercury

★ Undetectable levels of polycyclic aromatic hydrocarbons (PAHs)

★ Low peroxide values (PV). PV is a marker of rancidity; the lower the level, the better the oil. If the fish oil has not been stabilised with ingredients such as antioxidants, it can quickly become rancid and toxic

5

time to take action

A general word on **EXERCISE**

The exercise programmes in this chapter are all designed to increase your blood flow to problem fat spot areas and help transport fat away from the fat cells, and reducing the alpha 2 trap (pp20–21) in certain cases. Read this information before you get to grips with your particular fat spot later on in this chapter.

The most efficient way to lose weight is to combine cardiovascular exercise and resistance movements that challenge big muscle groups in both the upper and lower body. If you alternate upper and lower body exercises, your heart has to speed up, working at an elevated rate to pump enough fuel to the upper and then lower body muscles. This big effort helps to decrease body fat, increase lean muscle tissue and improve your body's metabolic rate to an optimal level to burn more calories.

WHAT IS INVOLVED?

For each fat spot, you need to warm up your muscles and get your heart pumping and blood flowing before undertaking alternate upper and lower body resistance movements. The beauty of these combined movements is that you work your whole body in one time-efficient session. Complete every session in the following sequence:

★ Cardio exercise (to warm up)
★ Upper body exercise 1
★ Lower body exercise 1
★ Upper body exercise 2
★ Lower body exercise 2
★ Cardio exercise (for some fat spots only)

See your individual fat spot section for your resistance exercises. They have all been specially chosen to ensure that you work the main muscles of your body with big movements, which will equate to you getting the best results.

Perform your exercise routine using either your own body weight or hand weights for added resistance, depending on your initial fitness level and familiarity with the movements. All the exercises can be done at home, outdoors or in the gym, and variations and ideas to progress individual exercises are provided within each fat spot section. In general, aim to work vigorously every time you exercise, but not so much that you physically can't perform another repetition. Research has shown that working yourself to 'failure' on a regular basis may have a negative effect on your body's hormonal response to exercise.

OTHER ACTIVITIES

In addition to following the six-week exercise programme for your particular fat spot, move your body as often as you can every day – by walking, climbing, dancing, lifting and stretching, for example. Also find some activities to do, preferably outdoors, that you find really enjoyable and uplifting. Together with your exercise sessions, what you are ultimately trying to achieve is an increased sense of energy and vitality and an optimal metabolic rate.

Any time spent in a calm environment or meditating with deep breathing will also help you to relax if your stress levels are high, and try to get at least eight hours' sleep at night so that your body feels as energised as possible.

THE RESISTANCE EXERCISES

See your individual fat spot exercise section for which exercises apply to you.
EQUIPMENT AT HOME and outdoors: use books (or a bag of books for a heavier weight), bottles of water of varying sizes, logs and so on as hand weights.
EQUIPMENT AT THE GYM or if you own equipment: barbell, dumbbells, weight plates, medicine ball, kettle bells, cable machine, lateral pull-down machine, assisted pull-up machine, bar fitted into a door frame, resistance band 1 (wrapped around something above head height), resistance band 2 (wrapped around an object above head height and your knees, and with your knees inside the band).

DEADLIFT

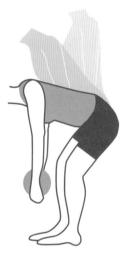

1 Stand with your feet positioned shoulder-width apart and place your hand weight(s), if using (bar, ball, dumbbell, bag, etc.), on the floor between your feet so that it is parallel with your toes.
2 Bend both knees until your thighs are parallel to the floor and let your arms hang between your legs. Grab hold of the weight(s) between your feet. Keep your chin parallel to the floor at all times and push your chest out.
3 Push through your feet and stand up tall while keeping your back straight. Then lower your hands to the floor, touching the weight(s) down gently, and repeat. Exhale as you stand and inhale as you lower.

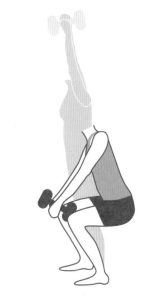

WOOD CHOP DEADLIFT

The wood chop deadlift is the same as the deadlift (overleaf), but with an additional arm movement incorporated:

From position **2** (the bent leg position with arms hanging between your legs), simultaneously elevate your arms in a swinging movement as you stand upright and lift your arms straight above your head (so you create a semi-circular pattern with your arms, if observed from side on). Do this using your own body weight or with additional weight, such as a medicine ball or hand weights, but start with light weights, as this is designed to be an energising movement.

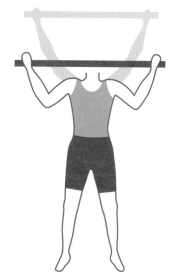

PULL-DOWN

1 Holding onto your hand weight(s), stand with your arms fully extended directly above your head and positioned slightly wider than shoulder-width apart. Use resistance band 2 for this exercise, if you prefer.

2 Pull down/lower the weight(s) and bend your elbows down and into your sides. Maintain a good posture with your chin up and shoulders back, and lengthen through the spine as you perform the movement.

3 Pause for a second, then return the band/weights back to the start position, keeping your shoulders down as you do so. Exhale as you pull down and inhale as you slowly return. Keep control of the band/weight(s) as you do so.

ALTERNATIVELY, perform a pull-up on a bar or fitted bar using your own body weight. An easier version of a pull-up is to pull yourself up from a seated position in the same way as above, but keep your feet on the floor and push through them to assist you.

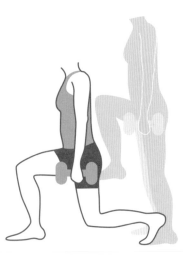

LUNGE

1 Stand in an upright position with your feet together. Hold some hand weights if you like.

2 Take a big step forward so that the shin of your stepping leg is vertical to the floor when you drop down. Drop your back knee close to the floor at the same time.

3 Push up and back to the original position for a static lunge or up and forward onto your front foot for a walking lunge. Alternate legs with each step. Maintain a good posture at all times with your body weight centred and your hips and shoulders parallel. Inhale as you drop down into the lunge and exhale as you stand up.

PRESS

1 Lie on your back in a supine position, ideally on pillows or a gym bench (so that your torso is slightly elevated off the floor and you can lower your elbows deeper to get a full range of movement).

2 Hold a weight in each hand. Extend your arms towards the sky, keeping your hands slightly wider than shoulder-width apart.

3 Lower the weights, bending your elbows but keeping your forearms pointing up, until your hands are either side of your chest and shoulders.

4 Hold this position for a second, then push the weights back up to the starting position (position **2**). Inhale as you lower the weights and exhale as you push back up. Keep your lower back in contact with the bench/floor/pillow at all times.

NOTE: A press-up is a version of a press using your body weight as resistance.

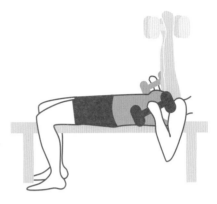

SQUAT

1 Stand with your feet shoulder-width apart with your weight evenly distributed across both feet so you feel rooted to the floor. Hold any hand weight(s) at shoulder height.

2 Bend your knees, push your bottom back and down, keep your chin parallel to the floor, and inhale.

3 Keeping your body upright, push through your feet as if pushing the floor away and stand up tall, exhaling as you do so.

SQUAT AND PRESS

1 Follow steps **1–3** of **SQUAT** for the legs, but hold your hand weight at chest level or, if using two single hand weights, at shoulder height.

2 As you stand up tall, extend your arms and push the weight(s) up so that when you are standing upright all the weight is above your head.

3 Return the weight(s) back to shoulder or chest height as you inhale.

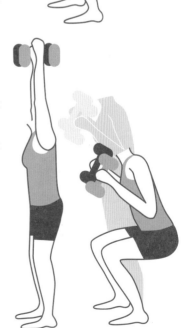

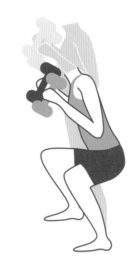

SUMO SQUAT

1 Stand with your feet wider than shoulder-width apart, toes pointed outwards, and hold your weight(s) at shoulder height. Keep your weight evenly distributed across both feet, your chin parallel to the floor and your body upright.

2 Bend your knees and lower your body down as deep as is comfortably possible by sitting back (as if sitting into a chair) and inhale.

3 At the bottom of your range push through your feet to return to your original upright position, exhaling as you do so.

ROW

1 Stand upright with your feet positioned shoulder-width apart. Use an overhand grip to hold your weight, if using, or stand in front of a bar or fitted bar. Hold onto it at mid-chest height and almost fully extend your arms.

2 Pull the weight/your body weight towards your chest/the bar, keeping a straight posture throughout. Pull your shoulders back, keep your elbows at shoulder height and squeeze your upper back, exhaling as you do so.

3 Inhale while slowly returning back to position **1**.

DOWNWARD DOG TO COBRA

1 Position yourself on all fours on the floor with your knees beneath your hips, your toes curled under so that they are gripping the floor and your hands beneath your shoulders.

2 Push your bottom up and back, extending your knees to straighten your legs, and inhale. Keeping your feet hip-width apart, push your heels towards the floor and straighten your arms. Lengthen the spine by pushing your chest down towards your toes. Hold this classic mountain position to get a good stretch through the body.

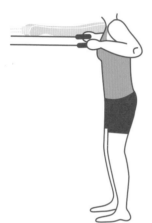

3 From downward dog, move into cobra: as you exhale, bend your elbows and allow your hips to come forwards and down so that your pelvis rests on the floor. Rest the tops of your feet on the floor. Then extend your upper body up at the end of the move by raising your head and chest as high as you can manage. Inhale and move back to position **1**.

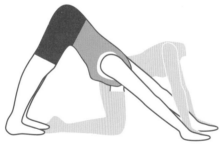

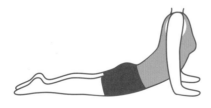

PECTORAL FLY

1 Stand with your feet positioned shoulder-width apart and hold a weight in each hand. Extend your arms out in front of your shoulders, palms facing each other with elbows very slight bent.

2 Move your hands away from each other to create a T shape with your body and arms (spread to the sides). Inhale as you do this, and maintain a good posture and straight spine throughout the movement.

3 Return to postion **1**, exhaling and keeping your arms straight with the elbows still very slightly bent.

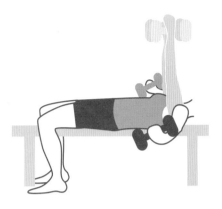

SINGLE ARM STANDING PULL

Repeat on the left side once you have completed these three steps:

1 Position a cable, or fix one end of a resistance band (resistance band 1), at head height. Hold the end in your right hand. Extend your right arm, step forward with your left leg and bend the knee. Your right leg will be behind you and almost straight (split stance). Bend your left elbow so your left hand is next to your left shoulder with the elbow held high.

2 Exhale and pull the resistance band back to your right shoulder. Straighten your left arm as you do so, bend your right leg and straighten your left leg so you rotate your body and your weight shifts.

3 Return to postion **1** with control, inhaling as you do so.

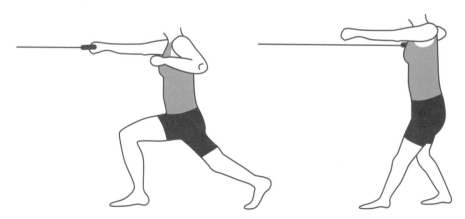

Love **HANDLES**

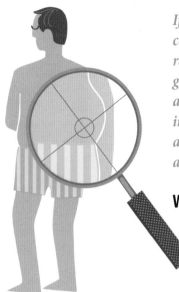

If you have love handles, you are more than likely experiencing the condition known as insulin resistance: when the body's cells fail to respond correctly to insulin in the bloodstream and refuse to allow glucose to enter cells, causing more and more insulin to be released and excess glucose to build up in the bloodstream. The other factor influencing your fat spot is alpha 2 receptors (pp20–21). The more alpha 2 receptors you have, the harder it is to lose weight in that area. So read on to bust your fat spot.

WHICH DIETARY HABITS CONTRIBUTE?

The types of carbohydrates we eat have a marked impact on our blood glucose levels and how hard our body has to work to maintain normal blood glucose levels. Foods that contain a high percentage of carbohydrate include cereals, grains, starchy vegetables (mainly root vegetables) and fruits. Carbohydrates are divided into two groups, simple and complex. Simple carbohydrates, which include glucose and table sugar, are found in high quantities in refined and processed foods like cakes, white bread, sweets and pastries. These simple carbohydrates are rapidly digested by the body and absorbed into the bloodstream, causing a sharp rise in blood glucose levels and resulting in a quick and excessive insulin response from the pancreas as it tries to mop up the excess blood sugars. The average western diet is full of these refined and processed foods.

WHICH LIFESTYLE HABITS CONTRIBUTE?

The two main adrenal hormones involved in dealing with stress and blood sugar control are cortisol and adrenaline (see box, p27). These hormones sharpen our reflexes and allow us to make quick decisions in dangerous situations. Stress increases the production of adrenal cortisol and this can result in insulin resistance, as cortisol prevents insulin from doing its primary job of transporting glucose into cells. I recommend a supplement on p91 to help your adrenals cope with the stress.

WHICH ENVIRONMENTAL FACTORS CONTRIBUTE?

Your family and peers are probably the largest environmental contributor to insulin resistance and the problems you now have with

DIGESTIVE PROBLEMS

In clinic I find that digestion may contribute to insulin resistance. Research shows that some of the body's natural immune chemicals, when activated, blunt the response of insulin to sugar. Factors include food sensitivities, leaky gut syndrome, infections such as candida, unfriendly bacteria and parasites. Seek appropriate testing and treatment if you think you might have one of these conditions.

sugar. If you grew up in a household where your family ate fresh, home-cooked, healthy foods, exercised daily and drank alcohol sparingly, and if your mum was super healthy during your pregnancy, the chances are that you have picked up these good habits and have no love handles. If the opposite was true, you probably have cuddly love handles. The argument of nature versus nurture does not apply in this case; nurture wins out almost every time.

What do you have to do?

1 Change your eating habits for the better by avoiding sugars and refined simple carbohydrates and opting instead for complex carbohydrates and foods that release energy slowly into your bloodstream. Keep reading to find out more about the highly effective eating plan you will undertake for the next six weeks.

2 Exercise. Movement is vital for life. It is now time to burn fat, get your circulation going and fine-tune your metabolism (see pages 92–93).

3 Optimising the way you use and metabolise carbohydrates is a large part of the solution. The modern nutritional supplements I recommend on pages 90 and 91 will optimise your energy levels and normalise the way your body uses carbohydrates and sugars. If you are worried about taking pills and potions, relax: the formulas I recommend are all tried and tested in my clinic.

FREE RADICALS

Our bodies burn glucose and oxygen to create energy, and during this process a number of unstable molecules called 'free radicals' are created. These molecules are highly reactive and cause huge damage to the body's cells. Free radicals are also produced during the detoxification of environmental toxins such as cigarette smoke, pollution and heavy metals. Normally the body is able to neutralise free radicals using natural dietary antioxidants such as vitamin C in oranges, lycopenes in tomatoes and the bioflavonoids in citrus fruits. If our antioxidant levels are low due to poor diet, stress or high exposure to environmental pollution, free radicals can damage our cells, increasing the rate at which we age. These bad chemicals also damage the insulin receptors on cells, making them less sensitive to the effect of insulin, which leads eventually to insulin resistance.

Your six-week **DIET** for love handles

To reduce your love handle fat, you need to reduce your intake of all simple sugars and refined carbohydrates. This is no easy task if you are used to the energy hit you get from a chocolate bar, for example. The basis for your diet for the next six weeks is the Mediterranean (MD) diet (pp70–75) so make sure you are comfortable with the MD principles and rules before embarking on the additional dietary changes (below) that are specific to this particular fat spot.

In addition to the MD diet, I also want you to adhere to two other dietary principles. There are two main scientific nutritional programmes in use that advocate a healthy, complex carbohydrate diet. They are the glycaemic index (GI) and glycaemic load (GL).

GLYCAEMIC INDEX

The glycaemic index rates how fast a certain food releases simple sugars (glucose) into the bloodstream. The higher the glycaemic index of a food, the higher your blood glucose levels rise after eating. A GI above 70 is considered high, a GI of 56–69 is medium and below 55 is said to be low. I have simplified this into 'good' GI (low and acceptable medium) and 'bad' GI (high) foods. To maintain constant blood glucose levels and avoid insulin resistance, I strongly advise you to limit your intake of 'bad' GI foods. See the box (right) for GI foods to avoid, and the box overleaf for those GI foods you can eat as part of your love handles programme. See also pages 96–97 for more information on GI foods.

THE GLYCAEMIC LOAD

The rating system known as the glycaemic load (GL) is a ranking system for the carbohydrate content of food based on its glycaemic index and portion size. Glycaemic load combines both the quality and quantity of a carbohydrate in one simple number. For example, maple syrup is a simple carbohydrate with a high glycaemic index, meaning it is converted into glucose quickly. But there may not be much maple syrup in your meal if you only add a dash of it to some plain yoghurt, so overall the dish will have a relatively low GL (even though the maple syrup has a high GI). A GL of more than 20 is considered high, 11–19 is medium and 10 or less is optimal for this diet. Obviously, foods with a high GI and a high GL are totally off-limits. To make things easy for you I have included the foods you should avoid in the same table (right).

DON'T EAT

As carbohydrates and sugars play a pivotal role in the creation of this fat spot, do not eat the following foods, which have a high GL and a bad GI.

UNHEALTHY GI AND GL FOODS TO AVOID

Alcohol (wine, beer, champagne, fizzy mixes, spirits)	Couscous	Puffed rice cakes
Baguette, white	Dates, dried	Raisins
Barley, pearl	Doughnuts	Rice noodles
Basmati rice, white	Fruit, canned in syrup	Rice, white
Biscuits, sweet and savoury	Fruit juices (except apple and grapefruit)	Rye crispbread
Black-eyed beans	Glucose	Split pea soup
Bread, white	Haricot beans	Table sugar (sucrose)
Buckwheat	Honey	Sultanas
Cakes and muffins	Malt and foods containing malt as a sweetener	Sweets
Chips (including French fries) and crisps	Millet porridge	All sweet snacks
Condensed milk	Muesli bars with dried fruit	Sweetened cereals
Cordials with sugar	Pasta, white	Sweetened fizzy drinks
Corn pasta	Peas, tinned	Udon (buckwheat) noodles
Corn tortilla	Potato, instant	Waffles
	Processed sweetened breakfast cereals	White flour
		Yams

✔ EAT

Watch your portion sizes. While a small handful of fresh grapes is fine, a whole punnet is a sugar feast. A single slice of rye bread works, but a few slices with breakfast and one with dinner is too much. Use your common sense, and eat lots of vegetables.

GOOD GI AND GL FOODS TO EAT (MAXIMUM AMOUNT PER DAY IN BRACKETS)

Agave syrup (1 tsp)
All-bran unsweetened
   cereal (1 small bowl)
Apple juice,
   unsweetened (150ml)
Aubergine
Beans, dried
Bread, mixed grain
   (1 slice), wholegrain
   pumpernickel (1 slice),
   wholemeal rye (1 slice),
   wholemeal sourdough
   (1 slice), wholewheat
   (1 slice)
Broccoli
Butter beans
Cabbage
Carrots, raw
Cashew nuts, raw (10)
Cauliflower
Chickpeas
Chillies
Egg fettuccini
   (1 small serving)
All fruits (see box, p73)

Fruit spread, 100%
   unsweetened (1 tsp)
Green beans
Haricot beans
Hummus (2 tbsp)
Kidney beans
Lentils, green
Lentils, red
Lettuce
Milk, skimmed
Muesli, no dried fruit or
   sugar (1 small bowl)
Mushrooms
Nut butter (1 tsp)
Oatcakes, whole oat (2)
Olives (10)
Onions
Quinoa (1 small serving)
Pasta, wholewheat
   (1 small bowl)
Peanuts, raw (30)
Peas, fresh green
Peas, yellow split
Pinto beans
Pitta bread, wholemeal
   (2 pockets)

Popcorn, no salt or
   sugar (1 small bowl)
Porridge, oat
   (1 small bowl)
Potatoes, new (3)
Red peppers
Soya milk, unsweetened
Sweetcorn, frozen
Tomatoes
Tomato soup, no
   added sugar
Vegetables (except those
   listed in 'Don't eat', p85)
Walnuts, raw (12)
Xylitol (natural sugar)
Yoghurt, natural,
   unsweetened

EAT PLENTY OF FOODS RICH IN ANTIOXIDANTS

Antioxidants help to prevent damage from free radicals and reduce insulin resistance. The Oxygen Radical Absorbency Capacity (ORAC) is a laboratory test developed in the US that shows the protective antioxidant levels of fruits, vegetables, juices, teas and other foods. I love this list (below), as you can quickly tell which foods are powerful health-protecting antioxidants; the numbers that follow them show how strong their antioxidant action is. (I have removed any high GI or high GL foods from the list.) Aim for as high an ORAC rating as possible, as this gives you more antioxidant power per meal. So, for example, add a teaspoon of ground cinnamon to your bowl of breakfast porridge or a few pinches of ground cloves to your herb tea, or find healthy dishes to make that include these foods as ingredients. Have at least two servings a day of the top antioxidant foods listed below, and include as many of the spices in your meals as you can.

ANTIOXIDANT-RICH FOODS

Cloves, ground 314,446

Cinnamon, ground 267,536

Oregano, dried 200,129

Acai berries, freeze-dried 161,400

Turmeric, ground 159,277

Cocoa powder, unsweetened 80,933

Cumin seed 76,800

Basil, dried 67,553

Curry powder 48,504

Sage, fresh 32,400

Ginger, ground 28,811

Pepper, black 27,618

Thyme, fresh 27,426

Marjoram, fresh 27,297

Goji berries, 25,300

Chilli powder 23,636

Flaxseed 19,600

Pecans, raw 17,940

Paprika 17,919

Tarragon, fresh 15,542

Ginger root, raw 14,840

Peppermint, fresh 13,978

Wild blueberries, fresh 9,828

Hazelnuts, raw 9,645

Cranberries, fresh 9,548

Red kidney beans, fresh 8,459

Black-eyed beans, raw 8,040

Pistachios, raw 7,983

Lentils, fresh 7,282

Blueberries, fresh 6,552

Plums, fresh 6,259

Blackberries, fresh 5,347

Garlic, raw 5,346

Raspberries, fresh 4,882

Almonds, raw 4,454

Red delicious apples, fresh 4,275

Strawberries, fresh 3,577

Broccoli, raw 3,083

Pears, fresh 2,941

Broccoli, cooked 2,386

Spinach, raw 1,515

Green tea, brewed 1,253

Cold-pressed extra virgin olive oil 1,150

MENU PLAN

My aim with this menu plan is to give you a broad idea of the kinds of meals you can prepare within the simple rules of my MD diet (below right). There are seven suggestions for every meal – a week's menu, in effect – if you want to adhere to this plan throughout the six-week diet, or adapt these suggestions as you become familiar with low GI and healthy GL foods.

I have also included a few snack suggestions. Have one in the morning and one mid-afternoon **ONLY** if you are feeling hungry. Snacking adds calories and calories add to your fat deposits.

BREAKFAST

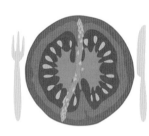

Choose from one of the following:

1 Oat porridge with one chopped fresh apple or pear
2 Muesli, unsweetened, with low-fat skimmed milk
3 Scrambled eggs on one slice of rye bread or toast
4 Oatmeal pancakes with fresh berries
5 Toasted oats with grated apple, dried cherries and almonds
6 Fruit salad with natural unsweetened yoghurt
7 A slice of rye bread, a teaspoon of nut butter and a teaspoon of fruit spread

LUNCH

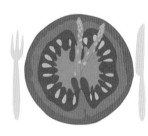

Choose from one of the following:

1 Tuna salad with two oatcakes and hummus
2 Grilled chicken and steamed vegetables
3 Bean salad, green salad and dhal (lentil soup)
4 Baked mushrooms with goats cheese and a side salad
5 Minestrone soup with cannellini beans
6 Avocado salad with chickpeas, tomato and roasted peppers
7 Spinach frittata

MAX'S TOP TIP

★ Consume healthy oils and proteins at every meal with your complex carbohydrates, as this will slow down the release of the carbohydrates into the bloodstream, thereby helping to keep your insulin levels steady.

DINNER

Choose from one of the following:

1 Vegetable and tofu stir-fry with cashews
2 Grilled lean beef, lamb burgers, pitta bread and lettuce
3 Stuffed peppers with green salad
4 Wholewheat spaghetti with aubergine, olive and tomato sauce
5 Grilled salmon with green beans, broccoli and ginger sauce
6 Skinless chicken on a bed of Puy lentils
7 Tomato and basil soup with two teaspoons of seeds

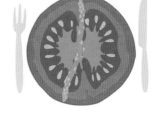

SNACKS

Choose from one of the following:

1 Sunflower seeds and apple slices
2 Slice of wholegrain bread and cashew nut butter
3 Fresh fruit – see box on p73 for portion control

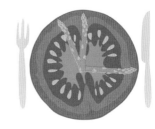

DRINKS

Drink warm herbal teas as a way of curbing your appetite and your need for oral stimulation. If you don't like herbal teas, drink warm water. Aim for six big mugs of herbal tea a day.

If you really can't manage without alcohol, you can have a single shot of vodka in the evening. One shot four times a week is your limit.

MD SIMPLE RULES

★ No sugar
★ Love your vegetables
★ High intake of fruits
★ High intake of legumes and beans
★ Regular intake of fish and seafood
★ Regular intake of wholegrain cereals
★ Very moderate intake of alcohol

★ Low intake of meat
★ Healthy fats, not no fat
★ Low intake of cows dairy produce
★ Include herbs and spices
★ Eat eggs
★ Enjoy nuts and seeds
★ Check your portion size
★ Eat with others

5

love handles

SUPPLEMENTS for love handles

Natural supplements help to balance your hormones and improve your sugar and carbohydrate metabolism. The nutrients needed to help you lose your love handles and control your blood sugars are those that I find are low in most clients I test.

DAILY MULTIVITAMIN AND MINERAL

Make sure that your multivitamin contains plenty of the vitamins C, B6 and B3, biotin and the minerals zinc, vanadium, calcium and selenium, as these are powerful antioxidants and also help to normalise insulin resistance. I suggest taking 1 tablet daily of a multivitamin that provides 100 per cent of the RDA (recommended daily allowance).

PURE FISH OIL

Take 3,000mg of pure fish oil a day or, if you are vegetarian, the same amount of organic, cold-pressed linseed oil (taken in capsule form or as oil drizzled on to food).

CINNAMON

Adding cinnamon to foods slows the rate at which the digesting food leaves the stomach and the resulting glucose enters the bloodstream. Just one teaspoon (1 gram) of this wonder spice lowers the gastric emptying rate by up to 35 per cent, according to research in the *American Journal of Clinical Nutrition*. Cinnamon is also a powerful antioxidant, helping to reduce the damage to insulin receptors by free radicals. If you don't like cinnamon or can't think of enough ways to include it to your diet, consider taking a daily supplement of 5g of cinnamon (*Cinnamomum cassia*). I take a teaspoon of organic cinnamon powder every day and wash it down with water. My only tip is not to breathe in when you take it!

CHROMIUM

We had a fabulous canteen at the college where I studied naturopathy in Sydney, Australia. It provided super-healthy food and plenty of salads and fresh fruit, but I preferred the amazing chocolate brownies. The only problem was that I got a massive sugar high followed by a crash in energy levels and ended up nodding off to sleep in lectures. My friend, who was

5

time to take action

about to graduate in naturopathy, took me aside one day and suggested that I was hypoglycaemic (I experienced particularly low blood glucose levels after my sugar highs), and that my body was not dealing very well with sugar. He suggested I take a chromium supplement, and in a matter of days my symptoms had disappeared.

Chromium is one of the most important nutrients for controlling blood glucose levels. The chromium content of food is greatly reduced by refining and processing so it is important to make sure you get enough. Your daily multivitamin and mineral will only contain a little so buy a chromium supplement that will top up your intake to 250mcg a day.

MAGNESIUM

Magnesium is an important mineral for numerous biological processes, including energy production and blood glucose control. Refining and processing food strips it of its magnesium content and magnesium deficiencies are common. Stress also has a major impact on magnesium levels. Once again, your daily multivitamin will contain only a little so buy a magnesium supplement that will top up your intake to 300mg a day.

ZINC

Hugely important with regard to supporting insulin function, zinc is necessary for the production of insulin and helps insulin to bind to receptors on the cells. A deficiency of zinc directly affects the action of insulin and interferes with proper digestion, creating deficiencies of the other important blood glucose control nutrients. Buy a zinc supplement to top up your daily multivitamin and mineral to 15mg a day.

GLUCOMANNAN FIBRE

This water-soluble dietary fibre improves blood glucose control and improves the action of insulin. It has the added benefit of reducing cholesterol levels in the blood. I suggest a dose of 10g a day, taken with plenty of water. Most good health food stores should stock it.

MULTI-VITAMIN 1 TABLET	FISH OIL 3,000MG	CINNAMON 1 TSP OR 5G	CHROMIUM 250MCG	MAGNESIUM 300MG	ZINC 15MG	GLUCOMANNAN FIBRE 10G

EXERCISE for love handles

This exercise programme is designed to energise you and help eliminate your love handles. Reread the general information and exercise descriptions (pp76–81) whenever you need a reminder of how to stay on track.

The resistance movements you will be doing are **PULL-DOWNS** and **PRESSES** for the upper body and **SQUATS** and **WOOD CHOP DEADLIFTS** for the lower body (pp78–81). These will work all the major muscles in your body and increase your circulation.

AIM

You need to use a full range of movement, working at a **MODERATE** intensity, almost to the point of each exercise being a stretch, and be very controlled with your breathing and tempo, moving and breathing to a ratio of 4–2 seconds. As your stress levels decrease and your fitness and energy levels improve, the resistance you use can become greater: increase the weights you use gradually and accordingly to keep you working within the same effort range, but don't increase the weight by more than 20 per cent from session to session.

Do every session in the same sequence **THREE** to **FOUR** times per week, preferably on **NON-CONSECUTIVE DAYS**.

CARDIO

Ideally you should walk or run, as this is the most natural way of performing cardio. Elevate your heart rate, though not to extreme levels, and work at a steady intensity for 5–10 minutes at 70–80 per cent of your maximum effort level so that you can still hold a conversation. Excessive cardio can place the body under further stress, so stick to the plan. Increase your cardio effort by no more than 10 per cent as you progress, and always check that you can still talk as you exercise. These steady increases will ensure that you do not overtrain your body, but continue to challenge it to the ideal levels for this fat spot.

OTHER ACTIVITIES

In addition to the exercise sessions, move your body as regularly as possible. Whenever the opportunity to do something physical presents itself, give it a go. Always take the stairs, not the lift, and walk to a local destination rather than drive. If you work at a desk, get out of your seat as often as possible and have a stretch. Anything medative and calming is also beneficial.

LOVE HANDLES EXERCISE PROGRAMME

Repeat exercises 1–5 in the same sequence two to three times		DURATION/REPS
1 GENTLE CARDIO (ELEVATE YOUR HEART RATE)	Running or brisk walking (alternatively, choose cycling, rowing or cross-training)	5–10 minutes (moderate intensity)
2 UPPER BODY EXERCISE 1	Pull-down ↓ 2 exhale ↑ 4 inhale	15–20 reps Rest for 30 seconds
3 LOWER BODY EXERCISE 1	Squat ↓ 4 inhale ↑ 2 exhale	15–20 reps Rest for 30 seconds
4 UPPER BODY EXERCISE 2	Press (or press-up) ↓ 4 inhale ↑ 2 exhale	15–20 reps Rest for 30 seconds
5 LOWER BODY EXERCISE 2	Wood chop deadlift ↓ 4 inhale ↑ 2 exhale	15–20 reps Rest for 30 seconds

KEY
↑ ↓ = direction of movement
3/2 = tempo (eg 2 or 4 seconds pushing, 2 or 3 seconds returning)
in/exhale = when to breathe

STOMACH Fat

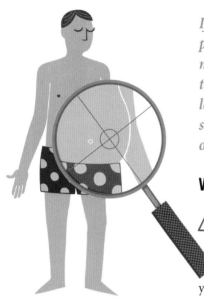

If you spend most of your life in 'flight or fight' mode – dealing with problems as though a lion has walked through your front door – it is not surprising you have a fat stomach. Unmanaged stress produces too much of the hormone cortisol (p15), which raises blood glucose levels. This, in turn, releases insulin, which stores the glucose as stomach fat. Alpha 2 receptors (pp20–21) can also affect fat storage on your stomach.

WHICH DIETARY HABITS CONTRIBUTE?

⚠ The main dietary culprit is an over-consumption of sugar-based calories, especially in the form of alcohol and refined (white) grains and flours: one 250ml glass of red wine contains around 180 calories, and an average pint has 230 or so calories. This may not sound a lot until you consider that two large glasses of red wine account for over 20 per cent of your daily calorie intake if you are a woman. The average glass of fruit juice contains 120 calories, a can of fizzy drink contains 145 calories and a butter croissant is over 250 calories. I could go on...

⚠ Coffee and other stimulants do not provide you with energy; rather, they stimulate your adrenals to produce adrenaline, making you feel as if you have more energy, until eventually you are exhausted.

WHICH LIFESTYLE HABITS CONTRIBUTE?

⚠ Modern life is all go, with too many deadlines, information overload and a diary full of chaos. Stress from any quarter will keep releasing the cortisol hormone into your system, which exacerbates your problem.

WHICH ENVIRONMENTAL FACTORS CONTRIBUTE?

⚠ Modern intensive farming methods have depleted the soil of much of its magnesium, an important stress-busting mineral that restores your beleaguered adrenal glands. Food-manufacturing processes also remove valuable vitamins such as B5 – another superfood for the adrenals.

⚠ Our exposure to electricity and electromagnetic radiation has increased by a phenomenal amount over the past two decades. These electrical appliances give off electromagnetic radiation fields, which spread

RELATED PROBLEMS

Stomach fat may increase your risk of a cardiac problem. Studies have found a link between increased waist circumference and heart attacks. In one study of 27,000 people from 52 countries, researchers found that as waist circumference increased, so did the risk of a heart attack. Those with the largest waists had close to double the risk of heart attack as those who had the smallest waists.

out into space indefinitely and carry alternating electric and magnetic vibrations. Electromagnetic (EM) pollution is a major stress on the body. Your health may be at risk from wireless emissions (wireless internet modems, mobile/wireless phones, cell and radio towers) and electromagnetic fields (computers, engines, inferior wiring, power lines).

Turn off and unplug all TVs, videos, computers and wireless routers when they are not in use. Turn your mobile phone off if you are not using it, especially in a long tunnel or if travelling on underground or subway trains. Don't have a TV in your bedroom and make sure that your alarm clock is battery-operated or placed away from your head. Don't have cables running under your bed, and unplug electrical items.

Another concern is that modern (DECT) digital cordless phones emit the same type of pulsed microwave radiation as (GSM) mobile phones. All DECT base units emit microwaves continuously as long as they are plugged in. If you must use a cordless phone, keep the base unit and extra handsets away from where you sit or sleep. Also think about buying phones that only transmit from the base when the handset is lifted, which cuts down on radiation.

What do you have to do?

1 Firstly, do less and chill out: anything that helps you to unwind and relax will mean less stress and less stomach fat. Rest also plays a major role in decreasing your cravings for calorie-dense foods such as chocolate; a recent study pointed out that even minor sleep deprivation increases our desire for comfort foods by 30 per cent. Try to get eight hours' sleep every night.

2 Change your eating habits for the better. In addition to following my Mediterranean (MD) diet principles, you will incorporate the specific elements of a glycaemic index (GI) diet. Foods with a low GI release sugar into the blood slowly, providing a steady supply of energy that leaves you feeling satisfied for longer so you're less likely to snack or overeat.

3 Follow a new exercise regime. Part of the reason for your expanded waistline is that you are too busy in your already busy life and have exhausted your adrenal glands. If you are getting up at 5am every day to spend an hour working very hard in the gym, you are further exhausting your knackered adrenals. Turn to pages 104–05 to find out how to change your routine.

4 By taking modern nutritional supplements that combine vitamins, minerals, medicinal herbs and other co-factors in synergistic formulations, you will nourish your tired adrenal glands and restore their balance and function. The formulas I recommend (pp102–03) are tried and tested and will put back what your hectic lifestyle has taken out.

5

stomach fat

Your six-week **DIET** for stomach fat

The best way to balance your blood glucose levels is to eat foods with a low glycaemic index (GI) that take time for the body to digest, thereby slowing down the amount of glucose entering your bloodstream at any one time. The basis for your eating plan is my Mediterranean (MD) diet (pp70–75); make sure you are comfortable with the MD principles and rules before embarking on the additional dietary changes (below) that are specific to this fat spot.

The **GLYCAEMIC INDEX** (GI) is a measure of the impact that food has on your blood sugar levels. Foods with a high, or unhealthy, GI are easy for the body to digest and quickly raise the levels of glucose circulating in your bloodstream. Foods with a low, or healthy, glycaemic index raise your blood glucose levels more gently over a longer period of time, as they take a while for the body to break down and digest.

A classic example of a high GI food is a can of sugary, fizzy soft drink. As you open the can and drink the contents, the sugar in the soft drink is quickly digested by the body and glucose enters your bloodstream in a rush, giving you an instant sugar high – followed swiftly by a sugar low and the need for your next can of sugary drink. On the other hand, the glucose generated by the body from wholewheat pasta or bread enters the bloodstream more gradually, thereby releasing energy over a longer period of time.

Elevated levels of glucose in the blood directly after eating high GI foods also triggers the release of insulin, and we know that insulin sweeps the excess glucose out of the bloodstream and stores it as fat. This makes it much harder to lose weight. Half the battle of stomach fat spot reduction is won by keeping your blood glucose levels stable in the face of stress-induced cortisol surges.

To make things simple for you, I have listed the foods you should avoid (right) while you are on this six-week diet. Do **NOT** feel free to ignore this 'Don't eat' food list. Then on the following pages I have listed foods with a low and medium GI that are suitable for this plan.

5

time to take action

X

DON'T EAT

HIGH GI FOODS	
DIETARY STAPLES	White breads, white pasta, white rice, white flour, biscuits, sweets, sweet snacks and confectionery
COWS DAIRY PRODUCE	Butter, cream, whole milk, full-fat yoghurt
BREAKFAST CEREALS	Processed breakfast cereals with added sugar, muesli with dried fruit
CONDIMENTS WITH ADDED SUGAR	Examples include mayonnaise, tomato ketchup and sweet chilli sauce (check all ingredients labels products for any mention of sugar)
FRUIT	Dried fruit of any kind (currants, sultanas, raisins, apricots, figs, dates and so on) fruit juices, high GI fruits (pineapple, mango, bananas, watermelon, cantaloupe melon and so on)
VEGETABLES	Potatoes
MALT	Malted processed cereals
BEVERAGES	Beer, lager, ales, stout, champagne, wine, mixers (for example, cola, tonic water), all fizzy drinks, cordials, fruit drinks, including concentrated fruit drinks to dilute to taste, coffee
SUGARS	Cane sugar, sucrose, glucose, fructose (as an ingredient), honey, chocolate, jams and marmalades, ice-cream, ready-made sauces

GI FACTS

★ High GI foods, which stimulate insulin surges, can cause people to eat up to 60 per cent more calories at the following meal: people who consume foods relatively high in glucose (such as white bread and pasta) eat an average of 200 calories more at the next meal than those who choose to eat low GI foods.

★ Recent scientific evidence shows that individuals who follow a low GI diet over many years are at a significantly lower risk of developing both type 2 diabetes and coronary heart disease.

★ In a study, rats fed on a high GI diet for 18 weeks were 71 per cent fatter and had eight per cent less lean (healthy) body mass than the low GI group of rats.

5

stomach fat

✓ EAT

FOCUS ON FRESH FRUIT AND VEGETABLES

Vegetables are the perfect foods to fill up on. The vegetables listed in the table (right) are guilt-free and antioxidant-rich. Snack on them, add them to your three main meals and generally over-indulge should you wish to. Make sure you also eat low GI fruits, but stay away from dried fruit, fruit juices and tropical fruits (see table, p97), as they are so high in sugar.

CHOOSE WHOLEGRAINS

Instead of buying high GI refined carbohydrates as your staple foods, choose wholegrain and wholewheat bread, wholewheat pasta and buckwheat pasta, wholegrain quinoa and brown rice instead.

AVOID COWS DAIRY PRODUCE

Choose goats or sheep dairy products – preferably low fat – rather than cows dairy produce, which is much higher in saturated fat. However, have as much low-fat natural unsweetened cows yoghurt as you like.

BUY MALT-FREE CEREALS

It's worth making your own muesli (toast enough oat, quinoa and barley flakes to make up a batch at a time, and add some nuts and seeds) or porridge, but if you do buy breakfast cereals, choose wholegrain cereals (such as 100 per cent corn flakes or puffed rice) with no added sugar. Read the ingredients labels to check that they really are free from malt and sugar.

TRY A HEALTHY SUGAR OPTION

Although sugar is something to be avoided, as are artificial sweeteners, you may use a low GI 'sugar' called xylitol. Xylitol is a natural sweetener derived from a compound, xylan, found in birch and other hardwood trees, berries, almond hulls and corn cobs. Xylitol looks, tastes and feels just like ordinary sugar, but has no aftertaste and has the same sweetness as sugar with only 60 per cent of the calories, so it doesn't elevate your blood glucose levels in the same way that ordinary sugars do. It can be used just like sugar in hot and cold drinks, on desserts and cereals and in baking. Have a maximum of one teaspoon a day. Ask for it at your heath food store or buy it online.

EAT MORE PULSES

Base your meals around beans, peas and lentils instead of high-GI potatoes and rice (especially the easy-cook variety). Pulses are slow-releasing and nutrient-dense and provide protein, fibre, iron, calcium, folate and soluble fibre (the fibre that helps to lower cholesterol levels).

EAT MORE FRESH NUTS AND SEEDS

Clients of mine, especially those looking to lose weight, often assume that as nuts are high in fat they should be avoided. This is not the case. Nuts are not only low GI and very filling, many are also great sources of essential fatty acids. Essential fatty acids are the only fats that can't be manufactured by the body and have to come exclusively from our diet. These good fats are important for weight loss and the maintenance of healthy blood glucose levels.

Eat all the foods listed in this table in moderation, except the vegetables.

GOOD GI FOODS	
VEGETABLES	Artichokes, green beans, asparagus, green apples, aubergine, spinach, bean sprouts, Swiss chard, broccoli, bok choy, Brussels sprouts, lettuce – all forms, cabbage, mangetout, cauliflower, mushrooms, celery, okra, chives, onions, leeks, kelp and nori seaweed, courgettes, radishes, cucumber, tomatoes, garlic, sprouts, peppers, kale Eat beetroot, butternut squash, carrots and sweet potato in moderation
PROTEIN	Eggs, fresh fish, skinless chicken, very lean red meat, tofu, tempeh
LEGUMES	Beans – black-eyed, butter, chickpeas, kidney, mung, pinto, soya
FRUIT	Apples, apricots, avocado, all berries, cherries, fresh figs, grapefruit, grapes, mango, nectarines, oranges, peaches, pears, plums, tangerines
NUTS AND SEEDS	Almonds, hazelnuts, walnuts, pecans, sunflower seeds, pine nuts, pumpkin seeds, sesame seeds, nut butters
OILS	Cold-pressed extra virgin olive oil
GRAINS	Amaranth, quinoa, brown rice, barley, buckwheat, millet, oats, 100 per cent wholewheat bread and pasta – wheat or rye, spelt
DAIRY	Skimmed milk, soya milk, oat milk, low-fat natural unsweetened yoghurt, buttermilk, kefir, low-fat goat and sheep dairy produce

★ No sugar
★ Love your vegetables
★ High intake of fruits
★ High intake of legumes and beans
★ Regular intake of fish and seafood
★ Regular intake of wholegrain cereals
★ Very moderate intake of alcohol
★ Low intake of meat
★ Healthy fats, not no fat
★ Low intake of cows dairy produce
★ Include herbs and spices
★ Eat eggs
★ Enjoy nuts and seeds
★ Check your portion size
★ Eat with others

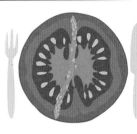

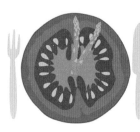

5

time to take action

MENU PLAN

You can either stick to this simple menu plan or experiment with it. Part of your long-term goal of eating well must be that you become expert in preparing healthy, tasty low-GI foods.

Aim to eat a quarter less food than you normally would. You can achieve this by chewing and tasting your food, which will make you feel fuller, sooner. Take your time and eat slowly. Eat only off a plate (so don't eat odd things from the fridge with your fingers, as you will end up eating more than you realise), sit down to eat, eat with a knife, fork or spoon and chew well. Try to eat until you are almost full, but never eat so much that you feel really full.

BREAKFAST

Choose one of the following:

1 One fresh pear and a small bowl of hot oat porridge made with skimmed milk, soya milk or water (add a few fresh berries to sweeten it if you like)

2 A small portion of scrambled eggs with smoked salmon (do not use cream or butter to make the eggs)

3 Fresh fruit salad – focus on fruits such as apples, pears, plums, cherries, peaches, citrus fruits and berries. Add a tablespoon of low-fat natural unsweetened yoghurt

4 A slice of wholegrain bread (containing nuts and seeds), thin avocado slices, tomato and some oily fish such as mackerel, salmon or kippers. Alternatively, use thin slices of turkey or chicken

5 Vegetable and egg frittata with chopped mushrooms, tomatoes, chopped chives or shallots. Add shredded turkey for additional protein

6 Banana smoothie with low-fat milk and cinnamon

7 Oat muesli with oat bran, sliced almonds, sunflower seeds, fresh wheatgerm and cinnamon

LUNCH

Divide your plate into three sections:

1 **HALF** of your plate must be a big raw mixed salad or lightly steamed vegetables. Include at least three different colour vegetables and dress the salad with cold-pressed extra virgin olive oil.

2 A **QUARTER** of your plate should include a whole grain of some sort. Try brown rice sprinkled with sesame seeds and mixed with a little tahini or wholewheat pasta with a sauce of chopped fresh tomatoes, torn basil leaves and finely diced garlic.

3 A **QUARTER** of your plate must contain a lean, low-fat protein. Choose from fresh grilled fish, smoked salmon, skinless organic chicken, organic eggs, tofu or lentils and add chopped fresh herbs to taste.

DINNER

Choose from one of the following:

1 Vegetable and bean soups (you may use a little vegetable stock in the recipe)

2 Cold gaspacho soup with a slice of wholemeal or wholegrain bread and a tomato and basil salad

3 Asian-style vegetable stir-fry with chicken, ginger and lime

4 Wholewheat pasta with fresh pesto with a fresh green salad and steamed vegetables

5 Vegetable ratatouille served with brown rice and sprinkled with sesame seeds

6 Tuna steak with a mixed bean and onion salad

7 Chicken and chickpea casserole

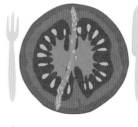

SNACKS

The art of keeping your blood glucose levels stable means that you need to snack between meals. This does not give you permission to have five huge meals a day: you should have three small, well-chewed meals and two good, low-GI healthy snacks.

Choose from the following:

1 A serving of lighty steamed vegetables drizzled with a little cold-pressed extra virgin olive oil and balsamic vinegar and a teaspoon of toasted pine nuts

2 A small selection of raw, unsalted nuts. Have a maximum of 12 nuts a day

3 Raw vegetable crudités such as celery, carrot sticks, broccoli and cauliflower florets with a little hummus as a dip

4 Low-fat natural unsweetened yoghurt with some pine nuts or berries

DRINKS

Have a large glass of water or a large mug of herbal tea as you wake up.

Drink warm herbal teas as a way of curbing your appetite and your need for oral stimulation. If you don't like herbal teas, drink warm water. Aim for six big mugs of herbal tea a day.

If you really can't manage without alcohol, you can have a single shot of vodka with fresh lime and soda in the evening. One shot four times a week is your limit.

SUPPLEMENTS for stomach fat

It's not only a good diet and stress-releasing exercises that will help to restore your adrenal glands. You also need nutritional intervention in the form of supplements to balance your cortisol levels and restore adrenal function.

DAILY MULTIVITAMIN AND MINERAL

Take a multivitamin that contains plenty of B vitamins and magnesium. I suggest 1 tablet daily of a multivitamin that provides 100 per cent of the RDA (recommended daily allowance).

PURE FISH OIL

Take 3,000mg of pure fish oil daily or, if you are vegetarian, 3,000mg of organic, cold-pressed linseed oil (taken in capsule form or as oil drizzled on to food).

ADRENAL DYSFUNCTION

Healthy adrenal glands secrete cortisol according to a daily rhythm. Rising cortisol levels help us to wake up in the morning, peaking at approximately 7–8am. Levels then drop through the day, often with a small dip between 3 and 5pm, to their lowest between midnight and 4am. Episodic spikes – eating food, for example – cause a small burst in cortisol levels.

There are three stages that the adrenal glands go through as you cope with physical and emotional stress. We are interested in stages 1 and 3, as they impact most on your stomach fat:

STAGE 1 'WIRED': you feel out of control, fearful, restless and tense
STAGE 2 'WIRED AND TIRED': you feel agitated, on edge and fatigued
STAGE 3 'TIRED': you feel mentally and physically exhausted

	YES OR NO
ARE YOU WIRED? Symptoms include feeling nervous, anxious, restless, tense, easily distracted, fidgety, irritable, 'out of control', hot flushes and food cravings, high blood pressure and melancholic depression.	
ARE YOU TIRED? Symptoms include being tired, apathetic, depressed, having numerous physical complaints, abdominal bloating, diarrhoea, chronic fatigue, impaired memory/learning, stomach obesity, reduced sex drive, tendency to feel cold and appear pale.	

IF YOU ARE WIRED, ADD:
REHMANNIA

Rehmannia (*Rehmannia glutinosa*) is the most important Chinese herb for disorders of the adrenal glands. I always use it in combination with schisandra (below). There isn't a standard recommended dose, but I recommend 50g a day. If you buy it online, buy from a reputable online health site (p157).

SCHISANDRA

Schisandra fruit has an adaptogenic action (it calms and strengthens the adrenals and the nervous system). Use a standardised extract of schisandra (*Schisandra chinensis*) containing 3–4% schisandrin, and aim to take 90mg a day.

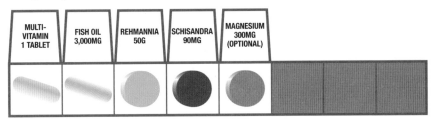

ADRENAL FORMULA

If you have stomach fat, you should also take a general adrenal support formula that covers most of the nutrients your adrenal glands need in order to function correctly and recover from exhaustion. Turn to resources (p157) for more details.

IF YOU ARE TIRED, ADD:
ASIAN GINSENG

The herb Asian ginseng (*Panax ginseng*) is an adaptogenic herb, a plant that helps the body to adapt and cope with physical and psychological stress, infections and environmental pollution. I suggest taking 400mg a day. Check on the label that it is standardised to a compound in the herb called ginsenosides.

RHODIOLA

A clinical study found that rhodiola (*Rhodiola rosea*) helped people with stress-related burnout, and numerous studies suggest it can help you adapt and cope better with stress. I suggest a dose of 300mg per day of an extract. Make sure the label says it is standardised to compounds rosavins and salidroside in the herb.

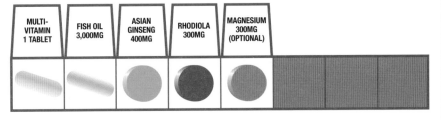

OPTIONAL SUPPLEMENT:
MAGNESIUM

Take 300mg of adrenal-nourishing magnesium to calm and feed the nerves.

IMPORTANT NOTE

⚠ Do not take these supplements during pregnancy or if you are breastfeeding.

⚠ Harmless changes in urine colour may occur if you use these products.

⚠ If you are taking medication, seek the advice of a medical practitioner or health professional first.

EXERCISE for stomach fat

Without question, exercise can reduce stress and make you feel and look much better. So now is the time to create vitality through movement, but without overly exerting yourself. Reread the general information and exercise descriptions (pp76–81) whenever you need a reminder of how to stay on track.

It is important to remember that you can't reduce stomach fat by doing endless abdominal crunches; working these muscles excessively could cause your stomach to get even bigger (by increasing the size of your abdominal muscles). The four resistance movements you will be doing are **SINGLE ARM STANDING PULLS** and **PRESSES** for the upper body and **WOOD CHOP DEADLIFTS** and **SQUATS** for the lower body (pp78–81).

AIM

You will be using a full range of movement, almost to the point of each exercise becoming a stretch, and be very controlled with the tempo and your breathing, moving and breathing to a ratio of 4–2 seconds. Together with the cardio these movements will help to energise you.

You need to work at a **MODERATE** intensity throughout. Using your own body weight or additional light weights as your resistance, work at the higher end of the repetition range, doing 15–20 reps for each exercise. As your fitness levels improve and your stress levels decrease, the resistance you use can become greater: increase your weights gradually and accordingly to keep you working within the same effort range, but don't increase the weight by more than 20 per cent from session to session.

As you don't want to over-stress your body, give yourself 30 seconds of controlled breathing recovery time between exercises.

Do every session in the same sequence **THREE** to **FOUR** times per week on **NON-CONSECUTIVE DAYS**, but don't stress if you miss a day.

CARDIO

Ideally you should walk or run, as this is the most natural way of performing cardio. Elevate your heart rate, though not to extreme levels, and work at a steady intensity for 5–10 minutes at 70–80 per cent of your maximum effort level so that you can still hold a conversation. Excessive cardio can place the body under further stress, so stick to the plan. Increase your cardio effort by no more than 10 per cent as you progress, and always check that you can still talk as you exercise. These steady increases will ensure that you do not overtrain your body, but continue to challenge it to the ideal levels for this fat spot.

STOMACH FAT EXERCISE PROGRAMME

Repeat exercises 1–5 in the same sequence two to three times		DURATION/REPS
1 GENTLE CARDIO (ELEVATE YOUR HEART RATE)	Running or brisk walking	5–10 minutes (moderate intensity)
2 UPPER BODY EXERCISE 1	Single arm standing pull (using cable or resistance band 1) ← 2 exhale → 4 inhale	15–20 reps Rest for 30 seconds
3 LOWER BODY EXERCISE 1	Wood chop deadlift ↓ 4 inhale ↑ 2 exhale	15–20 reps Rest for 30 seconds
4 UPPER BODY EXERCISE 2	Press (or press-up) ↓ 4 inhale ↑ 2 exhale	15–20 reps Rest for 30 seconds
5 LOWER BODY EXERCISE 2	Squat ↓ 4 inhale ↑ 3 exhale	15–20 reps Rest for 30 seconds

KEY

← ↑ = direction of movement

3/2 = tempo (eg 2 or 3 seconds pushing, 4 seconds returning)

in/exhale = when to breathe

OTHER ACTIVITIES

As well as doing your exercise sessions, find something enjoyable and playful to do, something that will allow you to forget all your stresses. Anything medative and calming is also beneficial.

BRA BULGE Fat

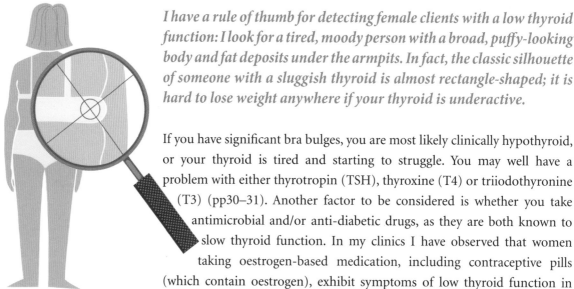

I have a rule of thumb for detecting female clients with a low thyroid function: I look for a tired, moody person with a broad, puffy-looking body and fat deposits under the armpits. In fact, the classic silhouette of someone with a sluggish thyroid is almost rectangle-shaped; it is hard to lose weight anywhere if your thyroid is underactive.

If you have significant bra bulges, you are most likely clinically hypothyroid, or your thyroid is tired and starting to struggle. You may well have a problem with either thyrotropin (TSH), thyroxine (T4) or triiodothyronine (T3) (pp30–31). Another factor to be considered is whether you take antimicrobial and/or anti-diabetic drugs, as they are both known to slow thyroid function. In my clinics I have observed that women taking oestrogen-based medication, including contraceptive pills (which contain oestrogen), exhibit symptoms of low thyroid function in spite of the fact that standard laboratory blood tests for a thyroid disorder usually shows no abnormal function (see box, right).

WHICH DIETARY HABITS CONTRIBUTE?

Goitrogens are naturally occurring substances in food that can interfere with the correct functioning of the thyroid gland and compromise the production of thyroid hormones. For this fat spot, limit your consumption of goitrogen-containing foods, which include broccoli, Brussels sprouts, cabbage, cauliflower, kale, kohlrabi, mustard, swede, turnips, millet, peaches, peanuts, radishes, soya beans and soya bean products, spinach and strawberries. However, if you do want to eat these foods, eat them cooked, not raw; research studies show that cooking these foods tends to deactivate the goitrogenic compounds. In the case of broccoli, as much as one third of the goitrogenic substance is deactivated when broccoli is boiled in water or steamed well. The foods listed above have many wonderful health benefits in areas other than the thyroid gland so do not cut them out of your diet if your thyroid is working well; these foods will not interfere with thyroid function in healthy people even when they are consumed on a daily basis.

Other dietary factors that may contribute to your fat spot include a deficiency of the mineral iodine in the diet, heavy metal toxicity, zinc and selenium deficiency and high alcohol intake.

SYMPTOMS OF A LOW THYROID FUNCTION MAY INCLUDE:

- ✔ Weight gain, especially round the middle and under the armpits
- ✔ Feeling cold, especially in the hands and feet
- ✔ Tiredness, especially after eating
- ✔ Brittle finger nails and hair and dry, flaky skin
- ✔ Poor memory and concentration
- ✔ Depression or anxiety or both
- ✔ Headaches/migraines
- ✔ Hair loss
- ✔ Fluid retention
- ✔ Constipation

5

time to take action

WHICH LIFESTYLE HABITS CONTRIBUTE?

⚠ Stress and the adrenals also play a part in influencing the thyroid hormones. During periods of internal stress (mental overexertion) and external stress (the pressure of events in the world that affect you), the adrenal glands produce more of the stress hormone cortisol and this in turn alters thyroid metabolism. The technical term is 'stress-induced thyroid imbalance' and it is characterised by lowered TSH production, which in turn causes a decline in T3 production. However, you can work on your stress levels; it is time to chill out.

⚠ A world-class athlete came to see me in my London clinic recently because she was cold, tired and feeling very run down. Excessive exercise can be very stressful on the body and may lead to thyroid problems, so I asked her to undertake a thorough thyroid test. It turned out that she had low levels of T3. She was under a lot of stress and permanently anxious because of a big event she was due to participate in. I explained to her that stress and anxiety may cause poor thyroid function and asked her to do some yoga and deep breathing each day. I also organised some daily supplements for her. Being disciplined, she did as I asked and took up the yoga and deep breathing. She rang a while later to say she was routinely breaking her personal best times and felt amazing. If you are feeling stressed, identify which issues could be causing this pressure and think about how you can shed these stresses in your life – or build in plenty of opportunities to relax more and unwind to counteract them.

STANDARD THYROID BLOOD TESTS

A standard medical blood test measures the levels of T4 and the thyroid-stimulating hormone TSH as a way of diagnosing low thyroid function. I have found several problems with this form of testing. Firstly, T4 is the precursor to the more active thyroid hormone T3 (p30). If there are any problems with the body converting T4 into T3, you may well have the symptoms of a low thyroid function despite having a normal T4 level. Secondly, the medical reference ranges for 'normal' thyroid function are very broad, and many of my clients have fallen within the 'normal' reference range despite having a blood level of T4 that is actually too low for them. Lastly, standard thyroid testing does not look at anti-thyroid antibody levels – an indication that you may have an autoimmune thyroid disease.

Each of these scenarios might potentially lead to patients not being diagnosed with a thyroid problem, even though they display typical symptoms and need naturopathic support.

Stop brushing your teeth with fluoride toothpaste. For decades, fluoride was used as an effective anti-thyroid medication to treat hyperthyroidism and was frequently used at levels below the current so-called optimal intake of 1mg per day. This is due to the ability of fluoride to mimic the action of thyrotropin (TSH). So buy a fluoride-free toothpaste from your local health food store instead. Filter your tap water, too, and research the effects of fluoride on human health online if you want to know more about this issue.

Other lifestyle factors that can impact negatively on the thyroid include a high alcohol intake, sustained sleep deprivation, major injury, illness and trauma.

BARNES TEST (ASSESSING HOW WELL YOUR THYROID IS FUNCTIONING)

1 Before going to sleep, place an oral thermometer within easy reach of your bed to test your basal metabolic temperature first thing in the morning.

2 Immediately upon waking, place the thermometer under your armpit and leave until the reading is ready to take (follow the manufacturer's instructions). It is important that you remain still and quiet in order to get an accurate reading; any movement will raise your basal temperature (your temperature when you first wake up).

3 Note the temperature and plot it onto a graph.

4 Try to do this at the same time each day.

5 Do tests on at least three consecutive days before you start your bra fat programme.

6 Do another test after six weeks to see how things have improved.

7 Your temperature should fall between the two thick green lines on the graph (between 36.6°C [97.9°F] and 36.8°C [98.2°F] – the normal range). If it doesn't, contact your health professional for a blood test. Start the programme, as it will be beneficial.

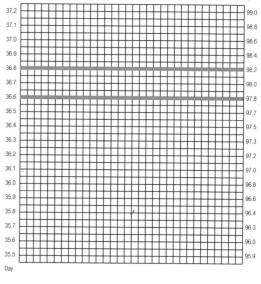

NB: Men can check their temperature on any three days. For women who are menstruating, your temperature is best measured on days two, three and four of your period.

WHICH ENVIRONMENTAL FACTORS CONTRIBUTE?

⚠ Scientific research is increasingly highlighting the close and often detrimental links between humans and our polluted environment. The quality of the air we breathe, the water we drink and the soil we grow our food in has a direct impact on the food chain, and therefore on us. We are regularly exposed to a large number of man-made chemicals, some of which are very toxic. Scientists have been aware for some time now that industrial chemicals are a source of concern with regards to human health, as they disrupt endocrine function (which is why these chemicals are also known as endocrine disruptors). Many studies also show that exposure to these environmental chemical pollutants may cause a subtle disruption of thyroid function. There is even evidence to suggest that exposure to chemicals such as PCBs (polychlorinated biphenyls, a man-made compound mainly used in electrical equipment), and dioxins (environmental pollutants) may even cause clinical hypothyroidism.

Minimise your exposure to these chemicals by limiting your intake of big oily fish such as tuna and swordfish and eat as much organic food as you can. Take a look at page 133 for more information on oily fish and PCBs.

What do you have to do?

1 This is a tough spot to get rid of and I want you to commit to a fairly tough diet plan and exercise regime. Watch how much you eat and re-read the diet section as often as you need to.

2 Take the natural hormone-balancing supplements I recommend. They are tried and tested formulas and are perfectly safe to take. Don't miss one dose of any of the supplements (pp114–15) for the full six weeks.

3 Follow your new exercise regime. All the exercises recommended have been carefully selected by a professional to get the best results (pp116–17).

4 Assess your thyroid function now with the Barnes axillary temperature test (taking your temperature under your armpit). This simple test (left) will help you to determine how well your thyroid is working.

5

bra bulge fat

Your six-week **DIET** for bra bulge fat

This diet is high in nutrients that will support your thyroid. Make sure that you are comfortable with the Mediterranean diet (MD) principles and rules (pp70–75) before embarking on the additional dietary changes (below) that are specific to this fat spot.

DON'T EAT

CHEAP AND RANCID OILS

A few weeks ago I read the headline, 'Standard supermarket oils can negatively affect thyroid health' in a respected newspaper. I totally agree. These are the oils we use every day and consume in commercially prepared and processed foods. However, these oils are extracted using chemical solvents and are then deodorised and stabilised with unnatural, thyroid-damaging chemicals. The most common source of these oils is soya bean oil, which is also a goitrogenic food (p106).

Cheap vegetable oils bought from a supermarket are not good thyroid food. All your oils must be extra virgin or virgin and cold-pressed. I recommend that you focus on olive oil, and please store all your oils in the fridge to stop them going rancid. Oils left in bright sunlight, exposed to air for a few days, or heated and re-used are most likely to be rancid (they will smell strange). Avoid these oils at all costs.

GOITROGENIC FOODS

Avoid the foods listed in the table below unless they are well cooked.

GOITROGENIC FOODS TO AVOID		
Broccoli	Millet	Soya bean and
Brussels sprouts	Mustard	soya bean products
Cabbage	Peaches	Spinach
Cauliflower	Peanuts	Strawberries
Kale	Radishes	Swede
Kohlrabi		Turnips

EAT

IODINE-RICH FOODS

The mineral iodine is a vital component of the thyroid hormones thyroxine (T4) and triiodothyronine (T3). Sea vegetables, especially kelp, are nature's richest sources of this important mineral. Although they look funny and may taste strange unless you cook them properly, they are major ingredients in Japanese and Korean food. Find some recipes that include kelp as an ingredient or borrow a Japanese cookbook from the library and experiment. I think of this as a great excuse to indulge my passion for sushi and California rolls.

SELENIUM-RICH FOODS

The enzyme that converts T4 into the active T3 contains selenium, which is also a potent protective antioxidant. Foods that are rich in this fabulous mineral include those listed here.

FOODS HIGH IN THE MINERAL SELENIUM		
Brazil nuts	Kelp	Salmon
Brown rice	Liver	Tuna
Chicken	Meat from grain-fed animals	Vegetables
Garlic	Onions	Wheatgerm
		Wholegrains

TYROSINE-RICH FOODS

Tyrosine is an amino acid – one of the building blocks for protein – and is another vital component of thyroid hormones. Natural food sources of tyrosine include the foods below.

FOODS HIGH IN THE AMINO ACID TYROSINE		
Almonds	Pumpkin seeds	
Avocados	Sesame seeds	
Butter beans		

MENU PLAN

My aim with this menu plan is to give you a broad idea of the kinds of meals you can prepare within the simple rules of my MD diet (below right). There are seven suggestions for every meal – a week's menu, in effect – if you want to adhere to this plan throughout the six weeks, or adapt these suggestions as you become familiar with the diet. Remember to eat sea vegetables – buy them from a health food store or a Japanese or Korean supermarket.

I have also included a few snack suggestions in case you have days when you are particularly hungry between meals and you feel that your energy levels are flagging. Have just one snack mid-morning, and one mid-afternoon.

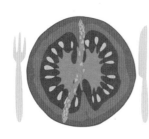

BREAKFAST

Choose from one of the following:

1 A slice of rye bread, a little non-hydrogenated margarine and pumpkin seed paste

2 Low-fat natural unsweetened yoghurt with wheatgerm and crushed Brazil nuts

3 Eggs, hummus and lean bacon

4 Oat porridge with almonds and sesame seeds

5 Fresh fruit platter with chopped almonds

6 Wholegrain muesli with Brazil nuts

7 Fresh fruit smoothie with wheatgerm, low-fat natural unsweetened yoghurt and a dash of agave syrup

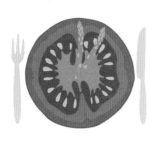

LUNCH

Choose from one of the following:

1 Vegetable soup with seaweed

2 California rolls with avocado, fresh tuna and nori seaweed

3 Brown rice stir-fry with green vegetables (although see list of which goitrogenic foods to avoid, p110). Add sesame seeds to flavour

4 White meat (turkey or chicken) with wholewheat bread/tortilla/pitta bread with lettuce and a drizzle of cold-pressed extra virgin olive oil

5 A salad of tomatoes and cucumber with a drizzle of cold-pressed extra virgin olive oil. Add some fresh fish and pine nuts and some freshly ground black pepper

6 Brown rice and chopped vegetable stir-fry with mushrooms and cold-pressed sesame oil

7 Grilled chicken with garlic and a crunchy side salad

DINNER

Choose from one of the following:

1 Grilled salmon and baked or roasted vegetables

2 Fish (salmon, prawns, halibut or snapper) with brown rice and aubergine

3 Salad with lettuce, tomatoes and peppers. Sprinkle chopped raw nuts or seeds over the top or add some cooked lean white meat

4 Grain-fed lean steak with steamed green beans and an onion and tomato salad

5 Fresh grilled tuna on a bed of brown rice, sesame seeds and a green salad

6 Miso soup with added seaweed

7 Fresh salmon sashimi and a Japanese salad of finely chopped vegetables drizzled with sesame oil

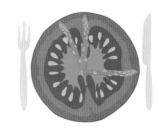

SNACKS

1 A handful of Brazil nuts, sunflower seeds (which are packed with selenium) and almonds

2 Fresh fruit such as apples, blueberries, avocados, mangoes, pears, cherries, plums, raspberries, cranberries and pineapples. Aim for one small bowlful a day

DRINKS

Drink a large glass of water or mug of herbal tea when you wake up. Drink warm herbal teas as a way of curbing your appetite and your need for oral stimulation. If you don't like herbal teas, drink warm water. Aim for six big mugs of herbal tea a day.

MD SIMPLE RULES

★ No sugar

★ Love your vegetables

★ High intake of fruits

★ High intake of legumes and beans

★ Regular intake of fish and seafood

★ Regular intake of wholegrain cereals

★ Very moderate intake of alcohol

★ Low intake of meat

★ Healthy fats not no fat

★ Low intake of cows dairy produce

★ Include herbs and spices

★ Eat eggs

★ Enjoy nuts and seeds

★ Check your portion size

★ Eat with others

SUPPLEMENTS for bra bulge fat

Natural supplements are necessary to balance your hormones and improve thyroid function. A common misconception is that you get all you need from food to stay healthy.

DAILY MULTIVITAMIN AND MINERAL

Your multivitamin should include B vitamins and copper, which are essential for the normal production of the thyroid hormones. Iodine is another essential nutrient for thyroid hormone synthesis (typical iodine deficiency signs include a metallic taste in the mouth and heavy mucous secretions). Make sure that your multivitamin has at least 150mcg of iodine per daily dose. This should be plenty, as long as you add some sea vegetables to your daily diet. I suggest taking 1 tablet daily of a multivitamin that provides 100 per cent of the RDA (recommended daily allowance).

PURE FISH OIL

Take 3,000mg of omega 3 rich pure fish oil or, if you are vegetarian, take 3,000mg of organic, cold-pressed linseed oil each day (taken in capsule form or as oil drizzled on to food).

SELENIUM

This mineral is essential for balanced thyroid hormone production. The enzyme that converts the thyroid hormone T4 into the more physiologically active T3 thyroid hormone is a selenium-containing enzyme. Without selenium this conversion cannot take place and so can lead to an under-functioning thyroid gland. Aim for 50–75mcg a day. Your multivitamin will no doubt contain some selenium, so add it all together and don't exceed 75mcg a day.

L-TYROSINE

Tyrosine is an amino acid and an essential component for the manufacture of thyroid hormones. The body must receive plentiful supplies of this amino acid in order for thyroid hormones to be produced effectively. Depression is clearly linked with low thyroid function, and I have found that clients with depression often have low levels of tyrosine. I suggest a dose of 1,000mg three times a day on an empty stomach.

IMPORTANT NOTE

⚠ Do not take these supplements during pregnancy or if you are breastfeeding.

⚠ Harmless changes in urine colour may occur if you use these products.

⚠ If you are taking medication, seek the advice of a medical practitioner or health professional first.

5

time to take action

VITAMIN D3

I prescribe this vitamin for all my thyroid clients and feel it is essential for good thyroid function and for thyroid hormones to be effective at a cellular level. I suggest 300mcg a day of vitamin D3. As this is a common vitamin deficiency, I suggest asking your doctor or health professional to test your blood levels. The doses needed to correct a deficiency are typically quite high, at 1,000mcg daily for eight weeks, so it is important that this is done under professional supervision.

ZINC

This is another essential mineral for optimising thyroid health. In a recent study of healthy people, thyroxin hormone levels tended to be lower in those people with a lower zinc intake. However, thyroxin levels increased after supplementing with zinc. There are many different zinc supplements available today and some are more easily absorbed by the body than others. I think one of the best sources is zinc picolinate. Aim for a total daily dose of 20mg. This will include the amount provided by your multivitamin and mineral.

HERBAL SUPPORT FOR OPTIMUM THYROID FUNCTIONING:
LIQUORICE ROOT

This amazing herb contains active flavonoids and a plant compound called glycyrrhizin. If you are feeling stressed or have just lived through a period of prolonged stress, liquorice (*Glycyrrhiza glabra*) will really help your thyroid by boosting your adrenals. Glycyrrhizin has been shown to inhibit the breakdown of cortisol in the body. Buy a capsule that is standardised to 25 per cent (75mg) glycyrrhizic acid and aim for a dose of 300mg a day. Do not exceed 400mg of glycyrrhizic acid a day, as it may elevate blood pressure.

GUM GUGGUL

Gum guggul (*Commiphora mukul*) is the sticky gum resin from the mukul myrrh tree and plays a major role in the traditional herbal medicine of India. Compounds in this resin support the conversion of the thyroid hormone T4 into T3 in the body. The dose I recommend is 300mg a day. Always use a standardised extract of 10 per cent guggulsterones.

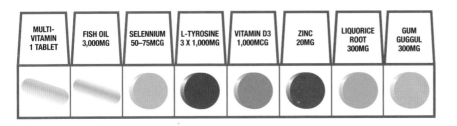

MULTI-VITAMIN 1 TABLET	FISH OIL 3,000MG	SELENNIUM 50–75MCG	L-TYROSINE 3 X 1,000MG	VITAMIN D3 1,000MCG	ZINC 20MG	LIQUORICE ROOT 300MG	GUM GUGGUL 300MG

EXERCISE for bra bulge fat

The aim here is to help bring your metabolism back to its most favourable level, de-stress you if you are feeling very fatigued and perform exercises that will energise you. It's time to start moving, but without overly exerting yourself, and creating vitality through movement. Reread the general information and exercise descriptions whenever you need a reminder of how to stay on track (pp76–81).

The resistance movements you will be doing are **ROWS**, **WOOD CHOP DEADLIFTS, DOWNWARD DOG** into **COBRA** and **SQUATS** (pp78–80). These will work all the major muscles in your body and increase your circulation.

AIM

You need to work at a **MODERATE** intensity throughout. Using your own body weight or additional light weights as your resistance, work at the higher end of the repetition range, doing 15–20 reps for each exercise. Use a full range of movement, almost to the point of an exercise being a stretch, and be very controlled with the tempo and your breathing, moving and breathing to a ratio of 4–2 seconds (except downward dog into cobra, which is 4–4 seconds). Together with the cardio, these movements will create a feeling of wellbeing and give you some much needed energy. When you notice an improvement in your strength and energy levels, steadily increase the repetitions you do or gradually add additional weights.

As you don't want to over-stress your body, give yourself 30 seconds of controlled breathing recovery time between exercises.

This session should be done in same sequence no more than **THREE** to **FOUR** times per week on **NON-CONSECUTIVE DAYS**.

CARDIO

If you have a trampoline at home or in your gym, use this for your cardio warm-up; walking or running are a good alternative. Elevate your heart rate, but not to extreme levels, and work at this steady intensity for five minutes. Work at 70 per cent of your maximum effort level so that you should still be able to hold a conversation while exercising. It is important to note that excessive cardio can actually increase cortisol levels and have a negative impact on your thyroid function, so stick to the limitations of this programme.

Increase your cardio effort by no more than 10 per cent as you progress, and always check that you can still talk as you exercise. These steady increases will ensure that you do not overtrain your body, but continue to challenge it to the ideal levels for this fat spot.

BRA BULGE FAT EXERCISE PROGRAMME

Repeat exercises 1–5 in the same sequence two to three times		DURATION/REPS
1 **GENTLE CARDIO (ELEVATE YOUR HEART RATE)**	Running or brisk walking (alternatively, choose cycling, rowing or cross-training)	5 minutes (moderate intensity)
2 **UPPER BODY EXERCISE 1**	Row ↓ 2 exhale ↑ 4 inhale	15–20 reps Rest for 30 seconds
3 **LOWER BODY EXERCISE 1**	Wood chop deadlift ↓ 4 inhale ↑ 2 exhale	15–20 reps Rest for 30 seconds
4 **UPPER BODY EXERCISE 2**	Downward dog into cobra ↓ 4 inhale ↑ 4 exhale	15–20 reps Rest for 30 seconds
5 **LOWER BODY EXERCISE 2**	Squat ↓ 4 inhale ↑ 2 exhale	15–20 reps Rest for 30 seconds

KEY
↑ ↓ = direction of movement
2/4 = tempo (eg 2 or 4 seconds pushing, 2 or 4 seconds returning)
in/exhale = when to breathe

OTHER ACTIVITIES

Move your body with a gentle flow on a daily basis and get outdoors whenever possible. Yoga will help you to practice controlled breathing while moving, and anything medative will also benefit you.

Bingo **WINGS**

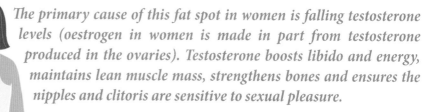

The primary cause of this fat spot in women is falling testosterone levels (oestrogen in women is made in part from testosterone produced in the ovaries). Testosterone boosts libido and energy, maintains lean muscle mass, strengthens bones and ensures the nipples and clitoris are sensitive to sexual pleasure.

WHICH DIETARY HABITS CONTRIBUTE?

⚠ High blood glucose levels decrease testosterone production, so you must keep your blood glucose levels in check by cutting sugar and refined carbohydrates from your diet. As you have detoxed and avoided sugar for a week, this shouldn't be as hard as it sounds.

⚠ You are not eating enough healthy, or 'good', fats. The healthy fats found in foods such as salmon, flaxseeds (linseeds) and avocados all contain excellent amounts of essential fatty acids (EFAs), and correct levels of essential fatty acids (pp72–73) are required for testosterone production.

⚠ You may be malnourished, even though you are probably eating more calories than you should and are most likely overweight. How is this so? We only have to go back a hundred years or so to compare the diets of our close ancestors with that of today's population. Our ancestors benefited from fresh, local and mostly organic produce. Farmers and gardeners then returned essential nutrients to the land by mulching, adding manure and compost and adhering to crop rotation, all of which serve to maintain soil quality and nutrient levels.

Modern foods are deficient in many essential nutrients for optimal health and hormonal function. Urbanisation has led to a move away from farm-fresh, natural foods. Chemical insecticides have replaced traditional methods of pest-control. Intensive cultivation and over-grazing have depleted the soil of valuable nutrients such as calcium, magnesium and the heart-protective mineral selenium. Transporting food long distances from farms to food-processing plants and supermarkets further depletes the nutrients. Vitamins A and C, for example, degrade with time, so the longer the distance from the farm to the table, the fewer there are of these nutrients. Vitamins B and C are building blocks for testosterone production and if they are not present in sufficient levels in your food, you may well have a testosterone problem.

WHICH LIFESTYLE HABITS CONTRIBUTE?

 Are you getting enough sex? Sex is a simple way to increase testosterone levels: as sexual intercourse depletes levels of testosterone, the body sends out signals to make more. A friend of mine who is a doctor recommends that her female patients make love at least once a week. Falling in love also increases a woman's testosterone levels.

 If you don't sleep well or for long enough, you will compromise your production of testosterone. Guard your sleep schedule, as you need deep sleep at the same time every night if at all possible. Getting adequate amounts of sleep is the best way to maximise testosterone production, as it peaks during the early morning.

 Stress suppresses testosterone production while relaxation increases it. Learn breathing techniques or meditation, listen to music, try aromatherapy or have soothing massages.

 Lack of exercise is another suppressor of testosterone levels. Weight-bearing exercise is a form of exercise that uses the body's own weight to place significant pressure on bones and muscles. This added weight causes the muscles to signal the cells for more energy and to request more testosterone to complete the exercise.

 Calorie-controlled diets or long-term consistent calorie restriction can cause lower testosterone levels. However, neither should you over-eat; it is vital that you eat less over the next six weeks and practice portion control.

WHICH ENVIRONMENTAL FACTORS CONTRIBUTE?

This is the one fat spot that does not have any major environmental factors, other than modern food production methods.

What do you have to do?

1 Increase your energy and vitality by following all aspects of this programme.

2 Feel alive and sexy again. You don't need to be in a relationship; thinking of yourself as a vital and sexy woman is just as effective.

3 Follow a weight-bearing exercise regime. See pages 126–27 for more information.

4 Take the nutritional supplements I suggest (pp124–25) to optimise your testosterone metabolism.

Your six-week **DIET** for bingo wings

Your bingo wings diet will be rich in healthy fats and lean protein. The basis for your diet plan is my Mediterranean (MD) diet so please make sure that you are comfortable with all the MD principles and rules (pp70–75) before embarking on the additional dietary changes (below) that are specific to this fat spot.

DON'T EAT

REFINED CARBOHYDRATES

For the next six weeks, do not eat any of the following:

CARBOHYDRATES TO AVOID		
White flour (eg, croissants, bread and cake)	Sweets	White pasta
	White rice	Sugary or fizzy drinks
Biscuits	White bread	Alcohol

SUGAR AND HIDDEN SUGARS

Listed below are some of the different ways sugar is labelled. Always read your food labels and keep a sharp lookout for any foods that contain these products so you can avoid them. (Artificial sweeteners such as saccharine and aspartame are all harmful to health and are also off limits on this programme.)

DIFFERENT FORMS OF SUGAR		
Brown sugar	Icing sugar (also called powdered or confectioners sugar)	Panocha (coarse Mexican sugar)
Corn syrup		
Demerara sugar		Rice syrup
Dextrose	Lactose	Sucrose
Fructose	Malt	Sugar (granulated and caster)
Galactose	Maltodextrin	Treacle
Glucose	Maltose	Turbinado sugar (unrefined crystallised sugar)
High fructose corn syrup	Maple syrup	
Honey	Molasses	
Invert sugar	Muscovado or Barbados sugar	

EAT

HEALTHY FATS

Eat healthy fats and stay away from saturated animal fats. If you add oily fish, fish oil supplements, cold-pressed extra virgin olive oil and cracked linseeds (flaxseeds) or linseed (flax) oil to your diet, your testosterone production will be at a premium. For example, drizzle a little cold-pressed extra virgin olive oil and balsamic vinegar over your vegetables at mealtimes. This not only tastes good, it ensures that you include healthy fats in your meal.

TYPE OF HEALTHY FAT	FOOD SOURCE
MONOUNSATURATED FAT	Olive oil, avocados, nuts and seeds
POLYUNSATURATED FAT	Vegetable oils (such as safflower, corn and sunflower), nuts and seeds
OMEGA-3 FATTY ACIDS	Fatty, coldwater fish (salmon, mackerel, herring), linseeds (flaxseeds), flax oil and walnuts

You may want to look in your health food store for a vegetable oil product that contains a blend of omega 3, 6 and 9 essential fatty acids. This is an excellent way of ensuring you include all the right healthy fats in your diet. Use it as the basis of a salad dressing or drizzle a little onto a bowl of soup before you serve it.

CHOOSE WHOLEGRAINS

Keep your blood glucose levels in check by only eating wholemeal and wholegrain cereals: brown rice, brown pasta and brown bread.

INCLUDE PROTEIN

Eat protein at every meal. For example, have an egg for breakfast in addition to a small portion of oat porridge (watch your portions), or add protein-rich seeds to the porridge. Add a few nuts and seeds to your salads, and beans, tofu, lean white chicken meat or flaked white fish to your soups.

USE A NATURAL SWEETENER

Xylitol is a natural sweetener derived from a compound, xylan, found in birch and other hardwood trees, berries, almond hulls and corn cobs. Xylitol looks, tastes and feels just like ordinary sugar, but has no aftertaste and has the same sweetness as sugar with only 60 per cent of the calories, so it doesn't elevate your blood glucose levels as ordinary sugars do. It can be used just like sugar in hot and cold drinks, on desserts and cereals and in baking. Have a maximum of one teaspoon a day.

★ No sugar
★ Love your vegetables
★ High intake of fruits
★ High intake of legumes and beans
★ Regular intake of fish and seafood
★ Regular intake of wholegrain cereals
★ Very moderate intake of alcohol
★ Low intake of meat
★ Healthy fats not no fat
★ Low intake of cows dairy produce
★ Include herbs and spices
★ Eat eggs
★ Enjoy nuts and seeds
★ Check your portion size
★ Eat with others

MENU PLAN

My aim with this menu plan is to give you a broad idea of the kinds of meals you can prepare within the simple rules of my MD diet (left). There are seven suggestions for every meal – a week's menu, in effect – if you want to adhere to this plan throughout the six-week diet, or adapt these suggestions as you become familiar with the diet. Just make sure you have protein, healthy fats and wholewheat carbohydrates at every meal.

There are also a few snack suggestions in case you are particularly hungry between meals and that feel your energy levels are flagging. Have just **ONE** snack mid-morning and one mid-afternoon, and watch your portion sizes.

BREAKFAST

Choose from one of the following:

1 (Breakfast smoothie)

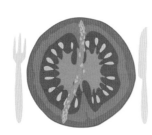

Berry smoothie

225ml milk or soya milk
200ml fresh orange juice
1 tsp or less xylitol
1 banana
175g fresh or frozen berries
   (blackberries, raspberries,
   strawberries)
1 tbsp whey protein powder
1 tbsp oil blend containing
   essential fatty acids (EFAs)

Place all the ingredients in a food mixer or processor and blitz until well blended and smooth. Serve and drink immediately.

2 Poached or boiled egg and smoked salmon on wholemeal toast
3 Quinoa porridge with a teaspoon of tahini stirred in and fresh berries
4 Mixed fruit salad with banana, figs and crushed almonds
5 Smoked mackerel and avocado on rye bread
6 Full-fat natural unsweetened yoghurt with some chopped fresh fruit and raw unsalted nuts
7 Omelette with tomato and red peppers

5

time to take action

LUNCH

Choose from one of the following:

1 Oven-roasted vegetables with steamed fish

2 Vegetable stir-fry with brown rice and kidney beans

3 Wholewheat pasta served with a fresh tomato and herb sauce and a mixed bean salad

4 Grilled chicken with steamed asparagus and a green salad

5 Lamb kebab (lean) with steamed broccoli and brown rice (once every 10 days maximum)

6 Turkey escalope, avocado and two slices of brown bread

7 Caesar salad with fresh vegetables and a boiled egg

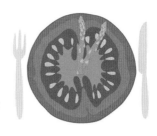

DINNER

Choose from one of the following:

1 Stuffed peppers with wild rice, feta cheese and cold-pressed extra virgin olive oil

2 Grilled chicken stir-fry with wholewheat noodles and sesame oil

3 Red kidney bean 'chilli con carne' with garlic, tomato and fresh herbs

4 Sirloin steak (very lean), brown rice and steamed cauliflower (once every 10 days maximum)

5 Oysters as a starter followed by steamed salmon with vegetables and brown rice

6 Omelette with broccoli, onion and grated goats cheese or halloumi

7 Beef and broccoli stir-fry in a ginger and garlic sauce (once every 10 days maximum)

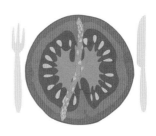

SNACKS

1 Fresh avocado slices (maximum ½ avocado a day)

2 Walnuts (maximum 12 a day)

3 Grilled chicken pieces

4 Fresh figs

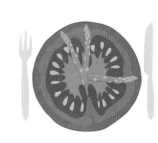

DRINKS

Drink a large glass of water or mug of herbal tea when you wake up.

Drink warm herbal teas as a way of curbing your appetite and your need for oral stimulation.

If you don't like herbal teas, drink warm water. Aim for six big mugs of herbal tea a day.

SUPPLEMENTS for bingo wings

I have recommended three supplements for you that are effective testosterone boosters. Don't be discouraged if your health food store does not stock some or all of these supplements; ask a shop assistant to order it in for you or go elsewhere (see resources, p157).

DAILY MULTIVITAMIN AND MINERAL

I suggest taking 1 tablet daily of a multivitamin that provides 100 per cent of the RDA (recommended daily allowance).

PURE FISH OIL

Take 4,000mg of pure fish oil or, if you are vegetarian, take 4,000mg of organic, cold-pressed linseed oil each day (taken in capsule form or as oil drizzled on to food).

NETTLE ROOT

A wonderful garden herb, nettle (*Urtica dioica*) can safely help increase testosterone levels in the body if used correctly and in the right amounts. In 1983, German researchers identified a constituent of nettle root that binds to SHBG (sex hormone-binding globulin, which binds to sex hormones in the blood, inhibiting their action), taking testosterone out of circulation in the body. In addition to inhibiting SHBG, natural plant compounds in nettle root inhibit aromatase, an enzyme that converts testosterone into oestrogen, thereby helping to preserve testosterone levels. Take 2 capsules of 300mg twice a day.

TRIBULUS

Tribulus (*Tribulus terrestris*) is one of the more commonly prescribed herbs for women with libido problems, as it is considered to stimulate testosterone levels. Buy tribulus that is standardised to 40 per cent saponins and 60 per cent protodioscin. Take 1 capsule of 300mg twice a day.

IMPORTANT NOTE

⚠ Do not take these supplements during pregnancy or if you are breastfeeding.

⚠ Harmless changes in urine colour may occur if you use these products.

⚠ If you are taking medication, seek the advice of a medical practitioner or health professional first.

5

time to take action

OATS AND GINSENG

A woman produces testosterone in her ovaries and adrenal glands. Modern life, and the demands placed on the average woman, can result in tired adrenal glands, which in turn impact on testosterone production. This is accentuated as a woman approaches and enters the menopause and her ovarian production slows: the tired adrenal glands need to take up the slack, which can lead to low testosterone levels. Fortunately, there is a class of herbs known as adaptogens that work to naturally rebuild adrenal function and restore hormonal balance. Foremost among the adaptogens are ginseng (*Panax ginseng*) and oats (*Avena sativa*). My favoured prescription is a liquid fresh plant tincture called ginsavena (the name may differ depending on where you live) that combines both ginseng and oats. I suggest a dose of 35 drops in water before breakfast and lunch. Do not take the tincture in the afternoon, as it energises the body and may subtly disturb your sleep pattern.

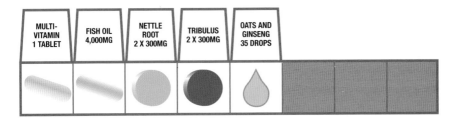

EXERCISE for bingo wings

This programme is designed to sculpt your body and develop your muscles while also relaxing you and decreasing your stress levels. It can be a tricky combination to master, but if you follow this programme and adhere to all the nutritional advice, you will be amazed with the results. Reread the general information and exercise descriptions (pp76–81) whenever you need a reminder of how to stay on track.

ROWS, **SQUATS AND PRESSES**, **DEADLIFTS** and **PECTORAL FLYS** (pp78–81) are the resistance movements you will be doing. These movements will work almost every muscle in your body.

AIM

You need to lift heavy weights well. Give yourself 60 seconds recovery time between each movement to allow you to put close to **MAXIMUM** effort into each exercise. Perform a repetition range of 8–12 reps, working pretty close to failure with each movement. For the first sequence, push yourself at about 80 per cent of your maximum effort level doing 12 repetitions, and for the second and third sequences do 8–10 reps, working at 90 per cent effort level.

Use your full range of movement so you work a larger portion of all the muscles activated. Attack the exercises while keeping perfect form, and move and breathe in a ratio of 3–1 seconds.

As your muscles develop your strength will increase, so increase the weights you use gradually and accordingly. Don't worry about turning into a body builder; this programme is simply designed to decrease your bingo wings and tone your body.

To avoid overtraining, give your body **TWO DAYS** to recover between sessions, so do a maximum of **THREE** sessions per week.

CARDIO

Finish each sequence with a short but high-intensity cardio blast followed by a good recovery (two minutes cardio, two minutes rest). Try sprinting up a hill, or do the same on a bike. The intensity depends on your condition, so if you are very unfit a brisk walk or climbing a flight of stairs may be sufficient to get you close to your maximum effort level. If you are in a gym, give the rowing machine or cross-trainer a go. As you get fitter, find a bigger hill or increase the resistance; consistently push yourself close to your maximum effort each time.

OTHER ACTIVITIES

Get a good night's sleep every night and incorporate gentle 'active recovery', which could be a walk in the park, some gentle yoga or an easy swim to help you recover and de-stress.

5

time to take action

BINGO WINGS EXERCISE PROGRAMME

Perform exercises 2–6 in the same sequence three times		DURATION/REPS
1 GENTLE WARM-UP CARDIO (ELEVATE YOUR HEART RATE)	Running or brisk walking (alternatively, choose cycling, rowing or cross-training)	3 minutes
2 UPPER BODY EXERCISE 1	Row ↓ 3 inhale ↑ 1 exhale	8–12 reps Rest for 60 seconds
3 LOWER BODY EXERCISE 1	Squat and press ↓ 3 inhale ↑ 1 exhale	8–12 reps Rest for 60 seconds
4 UPPER BODY EXERCISE 2	Deadlift ↓ 3 inhale ↑ 1 exhale	8–12 reps Rest for 60 seconds
5 LOWER BODY EXERCISE 2	Pectoral fly ↓ 3 inhale ↑ 1 exhale	8–12 reps Rest for 60 seconds
6 CARDIO BLAST	Running or brisk walking (alternatively, choose cycling, rowing or cross-training)	2 minutes at 80–90% maximum effort Rest for 2 minutes

KEY

↑ ↓ = direction of movement

3/2 = tempo (eg 1 second pushing, 3 seconds returning)

in/exhale = when to breathe

Big THIGHS AND BUTT

I hope you now have a clear understanding of how excessive oestrogen in the body may lead to inappropriate amounts of fat being deposited on your bottom and thighs, and also of the role of alpha 2 receptors in fat storage (if you need a quick refresher, reread pp18, 20 and 21). This section details other factors that may influence why you are fat here, and shows you how to bust your fat spot.

WHICH DIETARY HABITS CONTRIBUTE?

There are many dietary influences on this particular fat spot. Some have been proven by science while others, such as eating more fibre-rich vegetables, have been identified in my clinics. The focus for this section is on the modern western diet – I call it the SAD (standard Australian, American) or SUKD (standard UK) diet.

⚠ Fruit, vegetables, legumes and wholegrains are an abundant source of plant fibre, which binds to and excretes oestrogen from the body. It may come as no surprise to you that most modern diets, which predominate in refined white flour products rather than fresh fruit and vegetables, contain extraordinarily low levels of oestrogen-clearing fibre.

⚠ One of the key roles of the liver is to break down oestrogen and remove it from circulation. However, alcohol, pharmaceutical and recreational drugs, fatty bacon sandwiches and drinks laden with chemical preservatives and colouring agents can all hamper efforts by the liver to clear excess oestrogens that may enter the body from food and the environment.

⚠ Other contributing factors may include foods you are allergic to or have an intolerance to, excessive alcohol consumption and drinking bottled water from plastic containers. There is more on plastics later (p131).

WHICH LIFESTYLE HABITS CONTRIBUTE?

⚠ A prime suspect for me is contraceptive pills and HRT (hormone replacement therapy) that contain a high oestrogen component. If you are on an oestrogen-only pill, consider talking to your GP about changing to a low-dose combined pill (oestrogen and progesterone) or even a progesterone-only pill. Another option is to speak to your natural healthcare practitioner about alternatives to HRT and oral contraceptives.

time to take action

Many cosmetics contain chemicals that are reproductive toxins. Take time to review the lotions and potions you use every day and avoid any products with ingredients lists that include the word 'paraben'. Your health food or local organic store will sell skincare products and cosmetics that won't damage your health.

 Cigarettes and alcohol consumption damage hormonal control and production. Cutting down or cutting them out is an essential part of this programme.

Last, but certainly not the least important, is the fact that unrelenting stress sabotages hormone harmony. We all need to strive to do less and be more.

WHICH ENVIRONMENTAL FACTORS CONTRIBUTE?

Environmental pollutants are a modern phenomenon with a very modern effect on fat distribution. My particular focus is on xenoestrogens, chemicals that have a powerful oestrogenic effect (that is, they act in a similar way to oestrogen) on the body. They pass easily through our skin, and are found in many everyday products such as plastic containers, food cans, detergents, flame retardants, food, toys, cosmetics and pesticides. They are fat-soluble, non-biodegradable, dangerously toxic and leach into and contaminate the food we eat. Xenoestrogens are found in a wide range of substances, both natural and man-made, including pharmaceuticals, dioxins, polychlorinated biphenyls (PCBs), pesticides and plasticisers such as bisphenol A. These substances all harm the endocrine system.

What do you have to do?

1 Cut down levels of oestrogen: check your method of birth control and cosmetics and toiletry products, and avoid cigarettes, alcohol and stress.

2 Be ultra-conscientious about xenoestrogens. Eliminate any foods containing xenoestrogens and eat lots of cruciferous vegetables, which will help to modify your oestrogen metabolism.

3 Follow a new exercise regime. Turn to pages 138-39 to find out more.

4 Take the right hormone-balancing supplements that optimise oestrogen metabolism. In my clinic I use these natural treatments to help my clients restore function and optimise weight loss. The formulas I recommend (pp136-37) are all tried and tested.

Your six-week **DIET** for thighs and butt

To reduce your thigh and butt fat you need to reduce your intake of xenoestrogens and increase your consumption of cruciferous vegetables. Make sure you are familiar with the details of the MD rules (pp70–75) before embarking on the additional dietary changes (below) that are specific to this fat spot.

DON'T EAT
PROCESSED FOODS

Clinical evidence shows that processed foods high in sugar and fat contribute to hormone chaos. Eliminate refined white flour from your diet, too, and opt for wholemeal bread, pasta and grains instead.

COFFEE

Caffeine is a no-no, as studies show that two cups of coffee a day can increase oestrogen levels (see resources, p157).

FOODS THAT MAKE YOU BLOATED OR TIRED

Foods that have a negative effect on you are most likely allergenic in some way, and common food allergens disrupt hormones. The top allergenic food culprits are cows dairy produce, wheat bread, pasta and sugar. If your body rejects certain foods or finds them difficult to digest, stop eating them.

XENOESTROGENS

★ Many of the hormones used in modern farming methods include xenoestrogens. Eat organic meat and poultry instead, as these hormones are not used in organic farming. If organic food is too expensive, opt for 100 per cent grass-fed meat and dairy products.

★ Don't heat any food in a plastic bowl or with clingfilm on it in a microwave. When plastic is heated, chemicals can leach into the food being prepared. Common chemical culprits include xenoestogens such as BPA and phthalates and, according to the *Harvard Medical School Family Health Guide*, fatty foods like meat and cheese are especially susceptible to contamination. Use a glass or ceramic bowl instead, or heat food in a stainless-steel saucepan on the stove.

★ Don't eat any product that contains butylated hydroxyanisole (BHA) – a common xenoestrogen preservative in processed foods.

★ Minimise your consumption of canned food. It is estimated that over 85 per cent of tin cans are lined with bisphenol-A (BPA), a xenoestrogen, to reduce the metallic taste so often present in canned foods. BPA leaches into food when exposed to heat (pasteurisation) or acid. BPA is also present in many plastic baby bottles and food storage containers.

★ Don't drink liquids from plastic drinks bottles, as they most likely contain bisphenol-A (BPA). The xenoestrogenic chemicals present in the plastic bottles themselves will also leach into the drink if kept in a hot car or in the sun.

★ Water-treatment plants are not designed to remove hormonal pollutants, so agricultural and pharmaceutical run-off ends up in our tap water. To enjoy hormone-free water, I always recommend that my clients treat their water with a reverse-osmosis and carbon filtration system that will remove traces of BPA and other nasty elements from tap water (although they are expensive).

★ Non-stick pans are a potential source of xenoestrogens so go back to using iron or stainless-steel pots and pans and layer them with a thin film of olive oil to prevent sticking – an inexpensive, durable, and healthy alternative. Avoid aluminium cooking pots, as aluminium may play a role in the development of Alzheimer's disease.

★ Avoid plastics in the kitchen, especially soft plastics, as they contain many compounds that are considered to be xenoestrogens. Use glass or ceramic containers to store food.

★ Use clingfilm that does not contain DEHA, and replace the wrapped clingfilm on raw and ready-cooked meats and other foods as soon as you get home from the shops.

★ Also avoid:
★ PCBs (polychlorinated biphenyls) in paints and oils. Use natural paints instead.
★ All insecticides, pesticides and chemical lawn-care products at home. Find natural organic replacements at your local garden centre.
★ Sunscreen that contains 4-methyl-benzylidene (4-MBC), a xenoestrogen. Buy suncare ranges that are natural and chemical-free.
★ Creams, lotions, shampoos and bathing products containing parabens.
★ Synthetic flea shampoos, flea collars and flea pesticides for your pets and home.
★ Household cleaners, especially laundry detergents and fabric softeners, that contain xenoestrogens, as residues on clothing, towels and other items can come into contact with skin.
★ Air fresheners and insect repellents.

EAT

FOCUS ON FRESH FRUIT AND VEGETABLES

Aim to consume a variety of fibre-rich, organic seasonal fruit and vegetables, which contain a range of healthy phytonutrients (natural plant chemicals that have a positive impact on health). Eat at least two pieces of fresh fruit and four varieties of fresh vegetables every day (avoid canned or old produce). Frozen organic vegetables are also fine, but do make the effort to eat fresh fruit. Try to steam your vegetables or eat them raw, as boiling kills the healthy nutrients they contain, and always wash fresh produce before eating or cooking it to remove any surface contaminants.

CRUCIFEROUS VEGETABLES

Broccoli, cauliflower, Brussels sprouts, turnips, kale, green cabbage and mustard seed plants all possess unique phytonutrients that modify the way your body uses oestrogen. Eat three servings every day. These are all fabulous vegetables that contain a natural chemical, diindolylmethane (DIM), which is a major oestrogen-clearing phytochemical. When you chew raw or lightly cooked cruciferous vegetables, plant enzymes (substances that start a reaction) are activated, which allows DIM to enter your body. However, to get the most benefit from DIM over this limited six-week programme, you would need to consume very large quantities of raw cruciferous vegetables each day. To overcome this problem, I recommend you also take DIM as a dietary supplement for six weeks to boost oestrogen clearing (p136).

INCLUDE FIBRE IN YOUR DIET

Fruit, vegetables, legumes and wholegrains are an abundant source of fibre, which binds to and excretes oestrogen from the body, preventing the hormone from returning to circulation in the body and being re-used (and therefore exacerbating the problem of excess oestrogen).

EAT ORGANIC MEAT AND EGGS

If you can afford it, buy organic meat and eggs, as they are free from hormone residues that may include chemical oestrogen.

HAVE A DAILY DOSE OF GUT-FRIENDLY PROBIOTICS

Friendly bacteria assist in the clearance of oestrogen via the gastrointestinal tract. Probiotics can be found in the form of a live culture, such as live natural yoghurt with no added sugar, or as kefir in capsule form. Buy a reputable brand that guarantees up to two billion live bacteria per capsule.

EAT PLENTY OF WHITE FISH

Large predatory oily fish like tuna and swordfish may be contaminated with PCBs (a xenoestrogen that pollutes our oceans, see box, bottom) and mercury. Eat smaller oily fish that are not so high up the fish food chain, and eat more white fish than oily fish while on this diet. If you choose to eat big oily fish, keep your intake to just once a fortnight. Your local fishmonger or in-store fishmonger will be able to help you choose the right fish. I will also show you how to ensure that you have a sufficient intake of omega 3 oils (fish and linseed) in the supplement section (pp136–37).

VARIETIES OF FISH TO CHOOSE

OILY FISH	Anchovies, herring (bloater), kipper (herring), mackerel, orange roughy, pilchards (large sardines), salmon, sardines, swordfish (eat with caution), trout, tuna (fresh, eat with caution), whitebait
WHITE FISH	Cod, Dover sole, flounder, haddock, hake, halibut, hoki, John Dory, lemon sole, marlin, monkfish, plaice, pollack, pomfret (also known as butterfish), red and grey mullet, redfish (also known as ocean perch or rose fish), snapper (also known as red snapper), sea bass, sea bream, shark, skate, turbot, whiting

WHAT ARE PCBS?

PCBs, or polychlorinated biphenyls, are a group of man-made chemicals. They were used widely in electrical equipment and industrial processes until research revealed that they pose risks to human health, wildlife and the natural environment. PCBs are now banned, but PCB contamination remains widespread in the environment today because of the improper disposal of products containing the chemicals and by-products from the processes used to make such products.

PCB molecules attach, for example, to sediment particles, which may sink to the bottom of a river and are then eaten by tiny organisms. If small fish eat these organisms, they retain the PCBs in their body fat. This is repeated through the food chain to larger fish, birds of prey and humans – a process called bioaccumulation. PCB levels in top predators such as swordfish, lake trout and humans can be very high.

5

thighs and butt

★ No sugar
★ Love your vegetables
★ High intake of fruits
★ High intake of legumes
  and beans
★ Regular intake of fish
  and seafood
★ Regular intake of
  wholegrain cereals
★ Very moderate intake
  of alcohol
★ Low intake of meat
★ Healthy fats, not no fat
★ Low intake of cows
  dairy produce
★ Include herbs and spices
★ Eat eggs
★ Enjoy nuts and seeds
★ Check your portion size
★ Eat with others

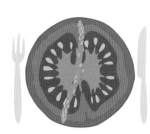

MENU PLAN

My aim with this menu plan is to give you a broad idea of the kinds of meals you can prepare within the simple rules of my MD diet (left). There are seven suggestions for every meal – a week's menu, in effect – if you want to adhere to this plan throughout the six-week diet, or adapt these suggestions as you become familiar with the diet. The only extra requirement is that you must eat three portions of lightly steamed cruciferous vegetables every day. Drizzle just a little cold-pressed extra virgin olive oil and balsamic vinegar or lemon juice over the vegetables, if you like, to make them taste delicious. If your work situation or daily routine means that you find it hard to eat a cooked meal at lunchtime, swap your lunch and dinner meals around.

I have also included a few snack suggestions in case you have days when you are particularly hungry between meals and you feel that your energy levels are flagging. Have just **ONE** snack mid-morning and **ONE** mid-afternoon.

BREAKFAST

Choose from one of the following:

1 Eggs, cooked as you wish (but not fried), with wholegrain bagel or toasted wholegrain bread rubbed with a little cold-pressed extra virgin olive oil

2 Wholegrain wrap with sweet peppers, chopped tomato, torn baby spinach, low-fat Feta cheese and a drizzle of cold-pressed extra virgin olive oil

3 Seasonal fruit with crushed raw cashews, almonds, pine nuts and a large dollop of low-fat unsweetened natural yoghurt

4 Baked apple with cinnamon and low-fat unsweetened natural yoghurt

5 Oat porridge with shredded apple and pine nuts

6 Boiled eggs with toasted rye bread

7 Cucumber slices, olives, white cheese (for example, halloumi, feta, cottage or goats cheese), torn fresh basil and wholemeal pitta bread

LUNCH

Choose from one of the following:

1 Grilled white fish or chicken with a variety of vegetables, especially cruciferous vegetables

2 Large dark green leafy salad with tomatoes, avocado, toasted pine nuts and a drizzle of cold-pressed extra virgin olive oil

3 Brown rice and vegetable stir-fry, which should include at least one cruciferous vegetable

4 Wholewheat pasta with a fresh tomato and olive sauce

5 Mixed bean soup and a tossed salad

6 Wholegrain couscous with lightly stir-fried vegetables

7 Broccoli soup with seeds scattered on top and a slice of wholemeal bread

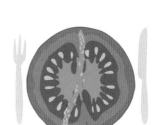

DINNER

Choose from one of the following:

1 A lightly steamed mix of cruciferous vegetables drizzled with olive oil and apple cider vinegar or balsamic vinegar

Plus **ONE** of the following:

★ Soup made with beans or legumes and cruciferous vegetables

★ Butternut squash soup

★ Vegetable ratatouille made with millet

★ Wholemeal bread, hummus, olives and a large colourful salad

★ Lentil soup with fresh herbs

★ Roasted curried cauliflower with brown rice

★ Brussels sprouts sautéed with pecans, fresh ginger and shallots

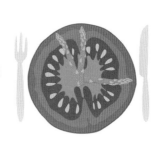

SNACKS

1 A small handful of fresh, raw nuts

2 Fresh tomato, sliced, seasoned and drizzled with a little cold-pressed extra virgin olive oil

3 Vegetable broth

DRINKS

Drink warm herbal teas as a way of curbing your appetite and your need for oral stimulation. If you don't like herbal teas, drink warm water. Aim for six big mugs of herbal tea a day.

5

thighs and butt

135

SUPPLEMENTS for thighs and butt

These nutritional supplements have been tried and tested in my clinic to help optimise the way oestrogen is used and metabolised. Take all the supplements listed here for the best result.

DAILY MULTIVITAMIN AND MINERAL

Take a high-quality daily multivitamin and mineral supplement that contains at least 50mg of each of the B complex vitamins (but 400mcg of B12) and 200IU of vitamin E, as these vitamins support oestrogen detoxification. I suggest taking 1 tablet daily of a multivitamin that provides 100 per cent of the RDA (recommended daily allowance).

PURE FISH OIL

Take 3,000mg of pure fish oil daily or, if you are vegetarian, 3,000mg of organic, cold-pressed linseed oil (taken in capsule form or as oil drizzled on to food).

DIM

The body breaks oestrogen down into 'good' and 'bad' oestrogen by-products, or metabolites. Diindolylmethane (DIM) is a natural compound found in cruciferous vegetables that promotes a more efficient manufacture of oestrogen: it promotes good oestrogen by reducing levels of 16-hydroxy (bad) oestrogen metabolites and increasing the formation of 2-hydroxy oestrogen (or good) metabolites. Many health benefits attributed to oestrogen, which include its ability to protect the heart and brain and its antioxidant activity, derive from these good metabolites. Obesity promotes the production of the bad oestrogen metabolites, as does exposure to environmental chemicals such as xenoestrogens. I recommend a daily dose of 200mg of DIM.

GREEN TEA

Green tea is a rich source of phytochemicals called catechins, and contains modest amounts of caffeine. Both catechins and caffeine have been found to increase fat metabolism; when consumed in combination – in a cup of green tea – they have an additive effect that is greater than either substance alone. Human studies have found that green tea, when drunk for an average of 12 weeks, resulted in weight loss or the prevention of weight gain after dieting. Enjoy a few cups a day without milk or sugar.

IMPORTANT NOTE

⚠ Do not take these supplements during pregnancy or if you are breastfeeding.

⚠ Harmless changes in urine colour may occur if you use these products.

⚠ If you are taking medication, seek the advice of a medical practitioner or health professional first.

5

time to take action

VITEX AGNUS CASTUS

An imbalance of the female hormones oestrogen and progesterone may lead to premenstrual stress (PMS). If you experience the following symptoms – all signs that you are oestrogen dominant – taking *Vitex agnus castus* will encourage your body to produce more progesterone:

★ Breast tenderness

★ Fluid retention

★ Irritability

★ Mood swings

★ Painful, heavy periods

I suggest taking a tincture, a fresh plant herbal liquid (one part herb to two parts alcohol). Take a 2.5ml dose every day in the morning.

CALCIUM D-GLUCARATE

This natural substance is found in many fruits and vegetables, especially apples, Brussels sprouts and broccoli. Oestrogen is metabolised in the liver by glucuronic acid through a process known as glucuronidation. It is then excreted in the bile unless an enzyme in the intestine called beta-glucuronidase breaks the oestrogen/glucuronic acid bond, allowing the oestrogen to be reabsorbed. Calcium D-glucarate inhibits beta-glucuronidase, allowing the body to excrete oestrogen before it can be reabsorbed and re-used. I recommend starting with a dose of 1,500mg and building up to 2,000mg over two weeks.

OPTIONAL SUPPLEMENT:
ISOFLAVONES

These are a type of plant-oestrogen found in soya beans, red clover, green tea, lentils and other legumes. The isoflavones genistein and diadzein (found in soya beans) have been shown in studies to be aromatase inhibitors. Aromatase, an enzyme found in the liver, is required for the conversion of male hormones such as testosterone into oestrogen. Aromatase inhibitors help to decrease the concentrations of oestrogen in the body. By inhibiting aromatase, the body produces less oestrogen and maintains a higher testosterone state. Aim for a supplement that gives you around 10–20mg a day of isoflavones. This dose is small, so you may need to break up the tablets to get the correct dose. Make sure you buy a product that is GMO-free (genetically modified soya is a no-go area).

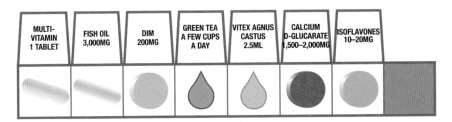

MULTI-VITAMIN 1 TABLET	FISH OIL 3,000MG	DIM 200MG	GREEN TEA A FEW CUPS A DAY	VITEX AGNUS CASTUS 2.5ML	CALCIUM D-GLUCARATE 1,500–2,000MG	ISOFLAVONES 10–20MG

EXERCISE for thighs and butt

Exercise is a key aspect of getting rid of your fat spot and optimising your sense of wellbeing. The cardio work and resistance movements in this programme literally work every muscle in your body to give effective fat-busting results on your thighs and butt. Reread the general information and exercise descriptions (pp76–81) whenever you need a reminder of how to stay on track.

You are going to work all the big muscles in your upper and lower body to get the biggest metabolic response. Your four resistance exercises are **PULL-DOWNS**, **LUNGES**, **PRESSES** and **SUMO SQUATS** (pp78–80). Don't worry about the possibility of increasing in size in these areas: muscle is extremely compact compared to fat; and women do not have the necessary testosterone levels to significantly build muscle mass.

AIM

Try to make every session one of **HIGH INTENSITY** and use moderately heavy weights for your upper and lower body movements. You need to consistently challenge your body during these sessions, working at a level of 80–90 per cent of your maximum effort level. As your fitness and strength increase and the weights you are using no longer challenge you to these levels, increase the weights you use gradually and accordingly to keep you working within the same effort range of 80–90 per cent.

Women generally respond better to higher repetitions of an exercise than men, so repeat each resistance movement 10–15 times. Keep your breathing controlled: inhale for three seconds and exhale for two seconds. Repeat exercises 2 to 6 in the same sequence **THREE** times for each session. The whole session should be performed **THREE** to **FOUR** times per week on **NON-CONSECUTIVE** days.

CARDIO

Ideally you should walk or run, as this is the most natural way of elevating your heart rate, but if you prefer to cycle, row or cross-train, that's fine. It is important to point out that excessive cardio can place the body under further stress and cause it to store more fat, so do not exceed the recommendations listed here.

OTHER ACTIVITIES

In addition to this exercise programme, freely move your body as much as you can, as often as you can, and find time every day to relax, meditate and practise some deep breathing.

THIGHS AND BUTT EXERCISE SESSION

Perform exercises 2–6 in the same sequence three times		DURATION/REPS
1 **GENTLE WARM-UP CARDIO (ELEVATE YOUR HEART RATE)**	Running or brisk walking (alternatively, choose cycling, rowing or cross-training)	3 minutes
2 **UPPER BODY EXERCISE 1**	Pull-down ↓ 2 exhale ↑ 3 inhale	10–15 reps Rest for 60 seconds
3 **LOWER BODY EXERCISE 1**	Lunge ↓ 3 inhale ↑ 2 exhale	10–15 reps Rest for 60 seconds
4 **UPPER BODY EXERCISE 2**	Press ↓ 3 inhale ↑ 2 exhale	10–15 reps Rest for 60 seconds
5 **LOWER BODY EXERCISE 2**	Sumo squat ↓ 3 inhale ↑ 2 exhale	10–15 reps Rest for 60 seconds
6 **CARDIO BLAST**	Running or brisk walking (alternatively, choose cycling, rowing or cross-training)	3 minutes at 70–90% of maximum effort Rest for 60 seconds

KEY

↑ ↓ = direction of movement

3/2 = tempo (eg 3 seconds pushing, 2 seconds returning)

in/exhale = when to breathe

5

thighs and butt

MOOBS (man boobs)

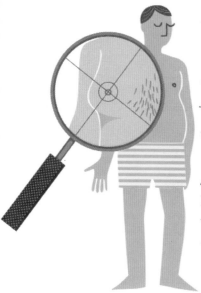

If you have moobs, the likelihood is that you have too much of the female hormone oestrogen in your system and not enough testosterone. The other reason may be due to an increase in the enzyme aromatose, an enzyme found in the liver that is responsible for the conversion of testosterone into oestrogen.

WHICH DIETARY HABITS CONTRIBUTE?

If you avoid cruciferous vegetables in your diet, you are missing out on the unique phytonutrients – which transform the dangerous hormone oestrogen into more benign forms – that they contain. Cruciferous vegetables include broccoli, cauliflower, Brussels sprouts, turnips, kale, green cabbage and mustard seed plants.

Do you like a beer? The hops in beer promote oestrogen in men. Switch to cider or even better still, drop all alcohol for a year to help your moobs disappear compeletely.

Do you regularly eat too much? If you are still eating and drinking like a growing teenager, **STOP**. Portion control is essential.

Xenoestrogens – man-made chemicals (see right) that mimic the action of the female hormone oestrogen with potentially feminising consequences – end up in the food we eat and the water we drink. Buy a good-quality water filter to eliminate xenoestrogens from your water supply and check with the manufacturer to make sure it does the job properly.

WHICH LIFESTYLE HABITS CONTRIBUTE?

I lay the blame firmly on our lack of adventures. When last did you do something that extended you physically and left you feeling vital and alive? Men need physical challenges so start planning something scary and daring. Undertake a 50-mile walk, climb a mountain peak, cycle across the country or run across a glacier; adventures make testosterone.

Testosterone is converted to oestrogen in the fatty parts of your body. The fatter you are, the more oestrogen you make. So start exercising, begin weight training, stop drinking, cut out junk food and eat less.

WHICH ENVIRONMENTAL FACTORS CONTRIBUTE?

⚠ One of the reasons for an excess of oestrogen in some men is environmental xenoestrogens or 'oestrogen-mimicking' molecules. Xenoestrogens are chemicals that have a powerful oestrogenic (they act in a similar way to oestrogen) effect on the body. They pass easily through our skin, and are found in many everyday products such as plastic containers, food cans, detergents, flame retardants, food, toys, cosmetics and pesticides. They are fat-soluble, non-biodegradable and dangerously toxic, and leach into and contaminate the food we eat. Xenoestrogens include a wide range of substances, both natural and man-made – pharmaceuticals, dioxins, polychlorinated biphenyls (PCBs), pesticides and plasticisers such as bisphenol A. To read about how to exclude them from your life, turn to pages 130–31. Look at the list of products that contain these chemicals and start avoiding them. You may want to write out the household foods and items that contain them and stick the list on your fridge to remind you.

⚠ Stress also damages testosterone levels, as cortisol, rather than testosterone, is produced in these periods of over-exertion. Late nights spent in front of the TV are not going to help you relax and de-stress either. Go to bed on time and wake up as it is getting light. The secret to a good night's sleep is undertaking effective exercise sessions through the week, eating early rather than late, keeping your bedroom dark as you sleep and turning off and unplugging all electrical equipment in your bedroom.

What do you have to do?

1 Eliminate xenoestrogens from your life.

2 Change your eating habits for the better. Follow the highly effective moob diet that I recommend for the next six weeks, and eat lots of cruciferous vegetables.

3 Using and building muscle improves testosterone production, so begin resistance training (using weights). Turn to pages 148-49 to find out more about how to exercise.

4 Sign up for an adventure today. Feel the fear and do it anyway. You will feel strong, virile and fighting fit by the time you have completed your challenge.

Your six-week **DIET** for moobs

This is the only fat spot diet plan that is not based on the Mediterranean diet. The diet I want you to follow instead is usually referred to as the 'paleolithic diet' referring to the Paleolithic, or Stone Age, era. It has changed little from the diet eaten by humans two million years ago. I don't advocate eating lots of red meat in the long term, so be aware that this protein-rich diet is designed to stimulate your testosterone production for the next six weeks only.

THE RULES ARE SIMPLE:

★ Only eat when you are hungry and not at set times of the day.

★ Eat lean cuts of meat from grass-fed animals, fresh fish, fruits, green leafy plants like rocket and spinach and lots of vegetables. The exact dietary mix is up to you. When I followed this diet I ate lots of barbecued chicken, masses of steamed green vegetables and a few pieces of fruit each day. You may be thinking that if you only eat protein and greens, how can you eat enough carbohydrates to fuel your training sessions? Vegetables contain carbohydrates so eat masses of vegetables every day. Try a handful of nuts and some carrots as a snack pre- and post training and don't use any of the carbohydrates and protein drinks sold in your gym.

★ Buy organic to avoid the chemicals modern farmers use.

★ Ensure that you eat healthy fats. Healthy fats, or essential fatty acids (EFAs), must be eaten as part of a balanced diet, since humans cannot make them. There are two families of EFAs: omega-3 and omega-6. Most of us get enough omega-6 EFAs due to a modern diet that is rich in grains and seeds and grain-fed animals, so I want you to focus on omega-3 EFAs. Sources of omega 3s are flaxseeds (linseeds), green leafy vegetables and cold water fish such as albacore tuna, sardines, Atlantic halibut and salmon, king salmon, herring, Atlantic mackerel and lake trout. However, some cold water fish have high levels of chemical pollutants, so take a quality fish oil supplement daily rather than overdosing on fish. Also, use plant oils such as avocado oil, coconut oil and cold-pressed extra virgin olive oil and limit your intake of butter, cream and fatty meats.

★ Add plenty of spices and herbs to your dishes, as this diet may seem a little bland otherwise. The natural plant chemicals in herbs and spices also contain powerful plant chemicals that energise and protect your body.

★ Practise portion control. Eat a third less than you normally would.

★ Don't eat grains, dairy products, beans, white and sweet potatoes, sugar, salt and all processed and junk foods (see box, bottom right). Include xenoestrogens in this list (pp130–31).

FOODS THAT TRIGGER FAT-BURNING HORMONES

The fat-burning human growth hormone (HGH), which is produced in the pituitary gland, decreases once you pass the age of 30, which is when your fat spot may start to grow. Research shows that HGH is triggered by several amino acids (proteins), arginine, glycine and tryptophan. So eat plenty of these foods, which are high in all three amino acids, over the next six weeks:

FOODS HIGH IN AMINO ACIDS	
Almonds	Oranges
Blueberries	Pecans
Brazil nuts	Pine nuts
Coconuts	Pumpkin seeds
Grapes	Sesame seeds
Hazelnuts	Walnuts
Mushrooms	Winter squash

All nuts and seeds need to be raw and sprouted (germinated). Simply soak them in warm water for 24 hours, making sure you rinse them thoroughly a few times, then dry and eat them. This is enough time to activate the seeds to create a 'living' food.

Interestingly, both HGH and testosterone are produced during very deep, or REM, sleep cycles so good sleep and deep rest are also vital.

INHIBITING AROMATASE PRODUCTION

Your diet and lifestyle are large factors in determining the amount of the enzyme aromatase (which converts testosterone to oestrogen) produced in your body. If you eat enough fruit and vegetables, you will have plenty of the flavonoids (a plant chemical) they contain, which have aromatase-inhibiting properties. Apples, cabbage, onions and garlic are good sources of quercetin, a powerful flavonoid, while the flavonoid apigenin is found in parsley, celery and chamomile (drink it as a tea). Flavonoids from flowers are found in significant amounts in bee propolis and bee pollen.

High levels of insulin, a big factor in weight gain and fat mass accumulation, may also promote the production of the aromatase enzyme. Keeping insulin levels under control by avoiding processed carbohydrates and junk foods results in lower levels of aromatase. Maintaining adequate zinc levels by eating red meat, pumpkin seeds and even oysters will also help to inhibit the production of aromatase.

EAT

★ Meat, chicken and fish
★ Eggs
★ Fruit
★ Vegetables, especially root vegetables, in particular carrots, turnips, parsnips, swedes (avoid potatoes and sweet potatoes)
★ Nuts such as walnuts, Brazil nuts, macadamia nuts and almonds (do not eat peanuts, as they are classified as a bean)
★ Berries such as strawberries, blueberries and raspberries

DON'T EAT!

★ Grains, including bread, pasta, noodles and cereals
★ Beans, including runner beans, kidney beans, lentils, peanuts, mangetout and peas
★ White potatoes and sweet potatoes
★ Dairy products
★ Sugar
★ Salt
★ Caffeine

5

moobs

143

MENU PLAN

This diet is very meat oriented and may feel quite brutal at times. It is very different from the average weight-loss diet. Feel free to look for recipes based on the paleolithic diet, but don't eat anything I have asked you not to eat (see box, p143) and always choose organic or grass-fed meat.

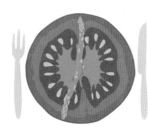

BREAKFAST

Choose from one of the following:

1 Beef tomato stew over steamed broccoli

2 Eggs, lean bacon and fried tomatoes. Use olive oil to cook your eggs and tomatoes. Do not fry them at a high heat

3 Grilled chicken breast, steamed spinach, diced raw carrots drizzled with cold-pressed extra virgin olive oil

4 Carrot salad with grated apple and meat leftovers

5 Fruit, including mixed berries, and grapefruit juice

6 Scrambled eggs with shredded chicken breast and a banana

7 Omelette with tomato, peppers and turkey slices

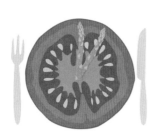

LUNCH

Choose from one of the following:

1 Omelette with fresh tomatoes and a small green salad

2 A piece of meat (any lean, organic meat will do) and a large salad

3 Mackerel or sardines, eggs and a mix of lightly steamed or raw vegetables and salad

4 Grilled salmon steak and lightly steamed vegetables

5 Chicken or tuna salad

6 Venison steak with fresh thyme and spring greens

7 Sardines, lightly steamed vegetables and a piece of fruit

DINNER

Choose from one of the following:

1 Whole chicken stuffed with herbs under the skin with a tomato salad and lightly steamed broccoli (save the leftover chicken for snacks)

2 Pork roast, lightly steamed cauliflower and broccoli and a tomato salad with pine nuts

3 Lean steak, oven-baked vegetables and lightly steamed broccoli

4 Steamed fish, asparagus and leeks

5 Lean steak and a large salad with nuts, cold-pressed extra virgin olive oil and tomatoes

6 Vegetable soup with chicken stock and coconut cream

7 Venison with lightly steamed broccoli, cabbage and carrot

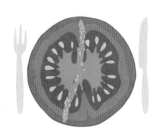

SNACKS

1 Nuts

2 Carrots

3 Fruit

4 Celery wrapped in air-dried ham

5 100 per cent meat sausages

6 Grapefruit

7 Olives

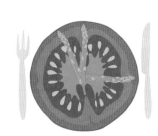

DRINKS

Drink water only, although you can also have raw coconut juice to add variety, if you wish.

If you have to drink alcohol, mix a vodka, real lime and soda and stay away from beer and wine.

MAX'S TOP TIPS

★ Remember that portion control is your new mantra. Simply eat one third less food than you normally would. If it helps you to practice honest portion control, try eating your food off a side-plate instead of a dinner plate.

★ Snack on protein when you feel hungry – for example, buy yourself some pre-cooked lean, skinless chicken breasts so that when you open the fridge in search of something to quieten your hunger pangs you have the optimal snack. Eat it with some raw vegetable crudités so you can keep up your vegetable intake.

SUPPLEMENTS for moobs

Dietary changes and tough exercise regimes give reasonable results on a moob programme, but nothing like the results I have seen when I recommend supplements to promote testosterone production. So a combination of diet, lifestyle changes and effective supplements is a winning one.

DAILY MULTIVITAMIN AND MINERAL

A good-quality daily multivitamin and mineral covers all nutritional bases and will ensure that you are not susceptible to a nutrient deficiency disease or dysfunction. I suggest taking 1 tablet daily of a multivitamin providing 100 per cent of the RDA (recommended daily allowance).

PURE FISH OIL

Take 6,000mg of a pure fish oil supplement or, if you are vegetarian, 3,000mg of organic, cold-pressed linseed oil (taken in capsule form or as oil drizzled on to food).

DIM

Diindolylmethane (DIM), a natural compound, is derived from indole-3-carbinol, which is found in cruciferous vegetables such as broccoli and cauliflower and is released when the body digests these vegetables. DIM promotes a more efficient oestrogen metabolism, causing levels of free testosterone to rise in the blood. The dosage I recommend for male moob loss is 200mg of DIM taken twice daily taken with food. Talk to your local naturopath or visit your health food store for more advice on purchasing a top-quality DIM supplement.

ZINC

Most men I see in my clinic are deficient in this vital mineral. Zinc is required for the metabolic activity of over 300 of the body's enzymes, some of which are involved in the metabolism of protein, carbohydrate, fat and alcohol. Poor zinc levels inhibit your general metabolism (the rate at which you burn food to make energy) and promotes the deposition of body fat. Studies suggest

IMPORTANT NOTE

⚠ Harmless changes in urine colour may occur if you use these products.

⚠ If you are taking medication, seek the advice of a medical practitioner or health professional first.

time to take action

that zinc is important for the production of testosterone. Zinc also inhibits the aromatase enzyme, which converts testosterone into excess oestrogen. Your multivitamin and mineral may contain up to 15mg of zinc; check the label first so that you know how much of a pure zinc supplement to buy. I recommend taking an additional zinc supplement that tops up your multivitamin dose to give you a total daily intake of around 30mg of zinc a day.

TRIBULUS

This is the herb that all the really big guys in my gym are taking. You may notice a change in your attitude in a matter of weeks – from slightly rounded and well breasted to a roaring cage fighter! In clinic, tribulus (*Tribulus terrestris*) is one of the more commonly prescribed herbs for men with libido problems, as it stimulates testosterone levels. Buy tribulus that is standardised to 40 per cent saponins and 60 per cent protodioscin. Take 1 capsule of 300mg twice a day.

CALCIUM D-GLUCARATE

This natural substance is found in many fruits and vegetables, especially apples, Brussels sprouts and broccoli. This supplement activity is largely due to the inhibition of beta-glucuronidase in the gut, which may allow the body to excrete hormones such as oestrogen before they can be reabsorbed. I recommend starting with a dose of 1,500mg and building up to 2,000mg over two weeks.

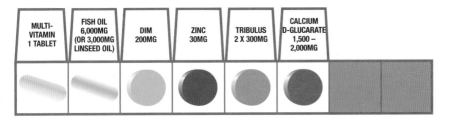

| MULTI-VITAMIN 1 TABLET | FISH OIL 6,000MG (OR 3,000MG LINSEED OIL) | DIM 200MG | ZINC 30MG | TRIBULUS 2 X 300MG | CALCIUM D-GLUCARATE 1,500 – 2,000MG | | |

EXERCISE for moobs

The point of this exercise programme is to boost your testosterone levels by developing your muscles and reducing your body fat; these sessions are designed to make you feel strong and alive. Reread the general information and exercise descriptions (pp78–81) whenever you need a reminder of how to stay on track.

You will be doing the following resistance movements: **PULL-DOWNS**, **SQUATS**, **PRESSES** and **DEADLIFTS** (pp78–79). These movements literally work every muscle in your body and increase your muscle mass, which will help you reach your optimal metabolic rate.

AIM

The emphasis is on lifting heavy weights well. Give yourself 90 seconds of recovery time between each set to allow you to put the **MAXIMUM** effort into each movement and enable you to lift big weights. Read the exercise descriptions carefully before you begin.

Work within a range of 6–12 repetitions for each movement, working pretty close to failure each time. The first sequence is a warm-up so do 12 reps, then for sequence two onwards work within an effort range of 80–100 per cent. You really need to push yourself during sequences three and four, so increase the weight you use and do just 6–10 reps. Allow 90 seconds' rest between each exercise.

Attack each exercise while keeping perfect form, moving and breathing with a ratio of 3–1 seconds. As you become more accustomed to the movements, your strength will grow so you will need to increase the weight you lift. However, don't exceed more than a 20 per cent increase in weights from session to session.

To give yourself enough recovery time, perform this session **THREE TIMES** per week on **NON-CONSECUTIVE DAYS** only.

CARDIO

Finish with a short, high-intensity cardio blast, followed by a good recovery (two minutes cardio, two minutes rest). If you are very unfit, a brisk walk or climbing stairs may be sufficient to get you close to your maximum effort. If you are in a gym, try the rowing machine or cross-trainer. Consistently push yourself close to your maximum each time. Note that it is pretty much impossible to go flat out for two minutes, so pace yourself while also pushing yourself.

OTHER ACTIVITIES

Organise physical adventures: go for a run in the park, or a wild run or wild swim. A good night's sleep and 'active recovery' such as some gentle yoga or a walk are also very important.

MOOB EXERCISE PROGRAMME

Perform exercises 2–6 in the same sequence three to four times		DURATION/REPS
1 GENTLE WARM-UP CARDIO (ELEVATE YOUR HEART RATE)	Running or brisk walking (alternatively, choose cycling, rowing or cross-training)	3 minutes
2 UPPER BODY EXERCISE 1	Pull-down ↓ 1 exhale ↑ 3 inhale	6–12 reps Rest for 90 seconds
3 LOWER BODY EXERCISE 1	Squat ↓ 3 inhale ↑ 1 exhale	6–12 reps Rest for 90 seconds
4 UPPER BODY EXERCISE 2	Press ↓ 3 inhale ↑ 1 exhale	6–12 reps Rest for 90 seconds
5 LOWER BODY EXERCISE 2	Deadlift ↓ 3 inhale ↑ 1 exhale	6–12 reps Rest for 90 seconds
6 CARDIO BLAST	Running (or brisk walking), cycling, rowing, cross-training or swimming	2 minutes at 80-90% maximum effort Rest for 2 minutes

KEY

↑ ↓ = direction of movement

3/2 = tempo (eg 1 second pushing, 3 seconds returning)

in/exhale = when to breathe

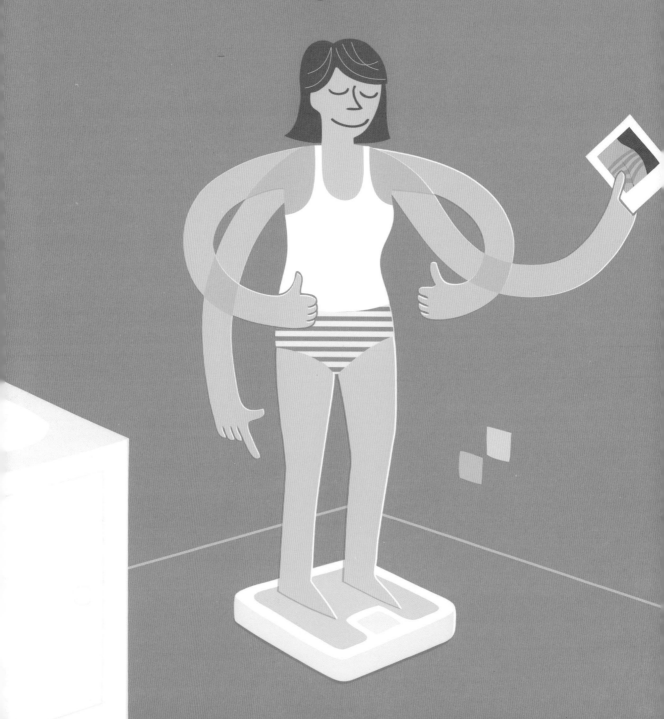

CHAPTER 6

Moving forwards

If you have successfully completed your six-week fat spot programme, well done! What you have achieved over the past few weeks is the beginning of a process of health restoration, not just the end of your fat spot programme.

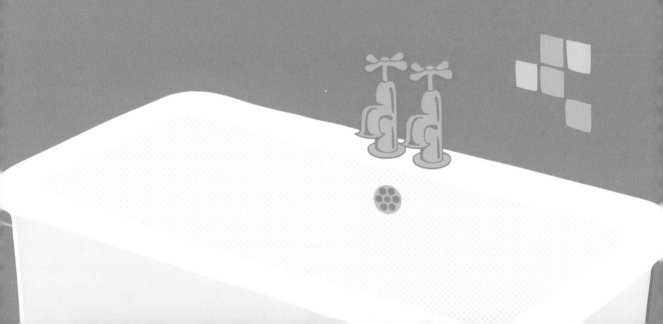

Moving **FORWARDS**

You have hopefully learned much about yourself and your body over the past six weeks, so don't spoil it now by stopping your new routine. I suggest that you assess the extent of your progress now that you are at the end of your fat spot programme.

You need to know how well you have done so do the full pinch test routine again (pp47–50) and compare the before and after measurements. Take another photo, too, so you can check your pre- and post-diet figures.

YOU ARE NOW FACED WITH THREE CHOICES:

1 Enjoy your well-proportioned body, and remain on the wonderfully healthy Mediterranean diet and keep up a regular exercise routine (based on your fat spot programme, if you wish)

2 Redo your fat spot

3 Tackle your next fat spot

WHY REDO THE SAME FAT SPOT?

If you haven't achieved your realistic goal, you may want to repeat the detox and six-week programme until you are happy with the results (there is no limit on the number of times you can do this). If you had an excessively large stomach or huge thighs, for example, a six-week programme may not make you as streamlined and super-lithe as you would wish, and your body may need more time to lose the extra fat.

DECIDING ON YOUR NEXT FAT SPOT

You started with your highest fat spot score, but your focus should now be on the fat spot that poses the most danger to your long-term health. Some fat spots are more dangerous than others and indicate a deeper, potentially more damaging imbalance. This is the list of six fat spots, starting with the most dangerous:

1 Stomach – cortisol

2 Love handles – insulin

3 Bra fat – thyroid

4 Moobs – testosterone

5 Bingo wings – testosterone

6 Thighs and butt – oestrogen

If you haven't already done so, you should repeat the pinch test before you decide to start a new fat-spot programme, as this is all about accurate observation.

How to **KEEP THE WEIGHT OFF**

If you are happy with the weight you have lost and feel that your body is back in proportion, here's how to avoid putting the weight back on. You are no longer on a diet, but there are several important points to remember.

1 SET YOURSELF A SIX-MONTH WEIGHT AND HEALTH GOAL Don't end up rudderless or drift back to old habits. Aim to stay the same weight and, if your fat spot grows, go back on the six-week programme. Don't be tempted to take just the supplements on their own, either.

2 FOLLOW THE SIMPLE RULES OF MY MEDITERRANEAN DIET

3 PRACTICE PORTION CONTROL We simply eat too much. Always eat one third less than you used to. Eating less has so many life-enhancing benefits, and Australian scientists have proved that eating less reduces your chances of getting cancer. If you are a compulsive overeater, get help. Work out what makes you overeat.

4 CHEW Digestion starts in the mouth so chew! Chewing also makes you feel full sooner and stops you from overeating.

5 DON'T DRINK WITH YOUR MEALS If you have to drink water with a meal, your food is too dry. Drinking water at mealtimes is just about the worst thing you can do, as it dilutes the concentrated digestive juices in the stomach that break down and digest your meal. A little wine is fine, but only one small glass.

6 DON'T EAT WHILE WATCHING TV Be aware of what you eat and how much you are eating.

7 STOP EATING WHEN YOU ARE ALMOST FULL – listen to your body.

8 EAT YOUR FOOD OFF A PLATE USING A KNIFE, FORK AND SPOON

HERE A FEW OTHER TIPS I HAVE PICKED UP OVER THE YEARS:

★ Don't use deep pasta bowls, as this results in big portions
★ Always measure your dried rice and pasta so you maintain a correct portion size
★ Don't hide evidence of your snacking – be embarrassed
★ Half of the food on your lunch and dinner plates should be vegetables
★ Don't load your plate; go back for more if you still feel hungry
★ Store fruit and vegetable snacks on the middle shelf of the fridge where you can spot them easily
★ Keep any sugary and fatty snacks at the back and top of the fridge
★ When eating out, only have two courses and remember that alcohol is almost a course in itself

6

moving forwards

EAT LESS, MOVE MORE CHECKLIST:

★ Walk to work
★ Walk to the shops
★ Ban the car
★ Have an active holiday instead of lying on the beach
★ Exercise each and every day of your life
★ Do your own gardening if you are lucky enough to have a garden

EAT LESS, MOVE MORE!

I have always thought that the basics of weight loss sound so simple. Eat less and move more. If only it were that easy. I had a giggle with a client recently. She was a little overweight and when I asked her about exercise she looked me in the eye and said that she did a lot of exercise – in fact, she went to the gym three times a week for one hour. She seemed rather pleased with her gym attendance until I told her that she spends less than two per cent of her week actively exercising. The point is that gyms are important, but movement is vital. If you sit on your backside for 98 per cent of your week then you are going to have a weight problem; I want you to **MOVE!**

EMPTY CALORIES VERSUS HEALTHY FOOD

I find that the best way to get the point across about avoiding empty calories to my clients is to give an example comparing a nutritious apple with an unhealthy chocolate bar:

1 CHOCOLATE BAR

50g
225 calories

NUTRITIONAL BREAKDOWN
Sugar
Saturated fat
Sodium

1 FRESH APPLE

100g
53 calories

NUTRITIONAL BREAKDOWN

Vitamins vitamin A, carotenoid, A retinol, A beta carotene, thiamine, riboflavin, niacin, vitamin B6, vitamin B12, biotin, vitamin C, vitamin D, vitamin E, folate, vitamin K, pantothenic acid

Minerals boron, calcium, chloride, chromium, copper, fluoride, iodine, iron, magnesium, manganese, molybdenum, phosphorus, potassium, selenium, sodium, zinc

Monounsaturated fats myristol, pentadecenoic, palmitol, heptadecenoic, oleic, eicosen, erucic, nervonic

Polyunsaturated fats linoleic, linolenic, stearidon, eicosatrienoic, arachidon, EPA, DPA, DHA

Other fats omega-3 fatty acids, omega-6 fatty acids

Amino acids alanine, arginine, aspartate, cysteine, glutamate, glycine, histidine, isoleucine, leucine, lysine, methionine, phenylalanine, proline, serine, threonine, tryptophan, tyrosine, valine, malic acid

Got it?

EATING TO LIVE, NOT THE OTHER WAY AROUND

If you are disciplined about food and have your eating under control, skip this section. However, if you are a comfort eater, do you eat, not because you are hungry, but for other reasons? Perhaps you are bored, fed up or depressed? You may even do it to cheer yourself up. If you are a comfort eater, ask yourself the following questions and answer them truthfully:

1 What emotions am I trying to suppress by eating?

2 What is the inner hunger I am trying to fill?

3 Am I eating out of boredom or frustration?

4 Does eating distract me from something else?

5 Am I eating in secret?

6 Why can I not stop after two chocolate biscuits?

7 Am I unable to refuse food?

8 When I eat, do I enjoy my food? Do I actually even notice I've eaten?

9 Do I eat up whatever is left – for example, on my children's plates – to avoid wasting food?

An occasional treat is good for you, but consistent comfort eating will lead to weight gain, and comfort eating while on a diet will undo all your good work.

CONSISTENCY AND YOUR ATTITUDE COUNTS GOING FORWARDS

A good relationship is built on trust and stands the test of time because both parties look out for each other and are consistent. In the same way your body needs you to have a better relationship with it. How can it trust you if one minute you are on a diet and the next you are raiding a sweet store? How can it trust you when you break all your exercise promises? Make your peace with your body and keep a positive, consistent attitude about it from now on.

GENERAL STEPS TO AVOID TOXINS IN YOUR FOOD, DRINK AND ENVIRONMENT

As I explained earlier, the environment we live in has become very polluted. Take steps today to reduce the amount of toxic chemicals that enter your body in the long term. Support organic agriculture and purchase as much organic food as you can afford. Support politicians that support a cleaner environment. Do not put chemical weed killers and insecticides on your lawn, pathways or plants. Use non-toxic cleaners at home, and try to manage insects and pests without contaminating your home. Use cosmetics that have little or no chemicals in them and use as few over-the-counter medications as you possibly can. Eat low on the food chain (in other words, eat a plant-based diet) and avoid animal fats, which contain the highest levels of dangerous chemical pollutants.

**SIX DAILY TOXIN
DETOX TIPS**

The following tips will help
you to eliminate waste and
reduce your toxic intake.

★ Drink plenty of water
  and herbal teas

★ Eat a variety of organic
  fruits and vegetables

★ Take your daily multi-
  vitamin and mineral and
  fish oil supplements

★ Eat lots of fibre

★ Exercise at least three
  times a week in addition
  to keeping moving. Use
  your fat spot exercise
  programme as a blueprint

★ Treat yourself to a sauna,
  steamy bath or massage
  whenever you need to
  – an important part of
  detoxing is being relaxed
  and relatively stress-free

STRESS MANAGEMENT - THE 'MUST HAVE' HEALTH TOOL

Stress can be a killer. If you live in a permanent state of stress you may end up sick or dead. I think that part of the reason we don't seem to take the potential effects of stress seriously is that we don't have a real awareness of just how dangerous it is to the human body. I am not talking about small stresses that annoy you, or about things that hassle you and niggle you. I am talking about the kind of stress that, if left unresolved, will damage your body and damage your mind. If for example, you are massively stressed out at work, with a huge work-load and no time for family and friends, then please be brave and address the situation.

You job is to de-stress your life. Down-size, down-shift and follow these tips:
1 Find someone to talk to about your stress levels. Don't bore a friend, as you will just add to their own stress. Find a kind and caring ear, even if you have to pay for it. Talk out your problems, your fears and your stress.
2 Do something each and every day that banishes stress, even if just for a little while. I have noted down some ideas, but you need to find one – or several – that helps you most:

✔ Walk   ✔ Play music and sing loudly
✔ Own a dog   ✔ Swim
✔ Cook   ✔ Cycle
✔ Yoga   ✔ Have a long, hot bath
✔ Meditation   ✔ Grow a herb garden
✔ Plant trees
✔ Read inspirational books

PLANNING THE FUTURE

I sincerely hope that you have achieved your goal and learned a lot about yourself and your health. These are my final four tips for your new future.

✔ Set a long-term goal for your health, weight and wellness
✔ Book your future seven-day detoxes into your diary. I suggest that you do one every six months (follow the detox in chapter four)
✔ Don't ever give in and grow or remain fat
✔ Love your body as it is – it's the only one you will ever have.

RESOURCES

RESEARCH PAPERS

pp26–27 *Journal of Diabetes Science and Technology* 2010
    May 1; 4 (3): 685–93

pp30–31 *Journal of Pharmacy and Pharmacology* 1998
    Sept; 50 (9): 1065–8

pp34–35 *Journal of Women's Health Gender-based Medicine*
    2000 Apr; 9 (3): 315–20

SUPPLEMENTS ONLINE

Nutricentre www.nutricentre.com
Bioforce www.avogel.co.uk
Biocare www.biocare.co.uk
Nature's Own www.natures-own.co.uk
Baldwins www.baldwins.co.uk
Nature's Plus www.naturesplus.com
Solgar www.solgar.co.uk

GENERAL ADRENAL SUPPORT FORMULAS

Anyone with stomach fat should also take an adrenal support
formula for 12 weeks. Below are four examples of quality
products I regularly recommend as general adrenal tonics,
and where to buy them online. Note: some formulas contain
raw bovine adrenal extract and as such are not suitable for
vegetarians or vegans.
Adrenal POWER Powder (www.adrenalfatigue.org)
AD 206 (Biocare www.biocare.co.uk)
AdrenoMax (Nutri www.nutri-online1.co.uk)
Adrenogen (Metagenics www.metagenics.com or Nutri www.
nutri-online1.co.uk)

OTHER WEBSITES

The George Mateljan Foundation http://whfoods.org
Dr. Udo Erasmus (oil) www.udoerasmus.com
www.max–tomlinson.com

FUNCTIONAL MEDICINE TESTING

See Benjamin Brown's monthly editorial 'Functional Medicine
Masterclass' in *CAM Magazine*, a complementary medicine
journal for health professionals in the UK.
See also www.timeforwellness.org

For more information on Genova and functional medicine
testing, see http://www.gdx.uk.net

INDEX

index

ACKNOWLEDGEMENTS

I would like to thank Paul Ranson BSc for creating and testing the exercise sessions; Benjamin Brown ND, consultant to the natural medicine industry, who has provided invaluable help on the supplements for each fat spot; and Dr Nigel Abrahams PhD FIBMS (Fellow of the Institute of Biomedical Science) and Scientific Director of CPA registered laboratory Genova Diagnostics Europe, who was kind enough to cast a critical eye over the theories behind my book.

Also to Susannah, my editor. Your patience and shining intelligence leave me speechless. Simply, thank you. Thank you, too, to Katherine for your design and and artworks, and to Jane and Borra: thanks for believing in me and supporting me on this journey of creation.

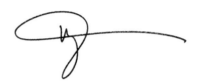

Paul Ranson has extensive experience in the fitness industry and has studied with the American College of Sports Medicine. He has also worked with Gary Ward, the founder of Anatomy in Motion, and has attended courses with Frank Forencich, the American-based human movement guru.

Editorial Director: Jane O'Shea
Art Director: Helen Lewis
Project Editor: Susannah Steel
Designer: Katherine Case
Illustrators: Nick Radford & Katherine Case
Production Director: Vincent Smith
Production Controller: Aysun Hughes

First published in 2011 by
Quadrille Publishing Limited
Alhambra House
27–31 Charing Cross Road
London WC2H 0LS

Text copyright © Max Tomlinson 2011
Exercise text copyright © Paul Ranson 2011
Illustration © Nick Radford 2011
Design and layout copyright © Quadrille Publishing Limited 2011

Cataloguing-in-Publication Data: a catalogue record for this book is available from the British Library.

ISBN 978 1 84400 820 9